American
Heart
Association.

Basic Life Support

PROVIDER MANUAL

ISBN 978-1-61669-768-6
Printed in the United States of America

First American Heart Association Printing October 2020
10 9 8 7 6 5 4

Acknowledgments

The American Heart Association thanks the following people for their contributions to the development of this manual: Jose G. Cabañas, MD, MPH; Jeanette Previdi, MPH, RN; Matthew Douma, RN; Bryan Fischberg, NRP; Sonni Logan, MSN, RN, CEN, CVN, CPEN; Mary Elizabeth Mancini, RN, PhD, NE-BC; Randy Wax, MD, MEd; Sharon T. Wilson, PhD, RN, FCN; Brenda D. Schoolfield; and the AHA BLS Project Team.

The AHA has published Interim Guidance to Health Care for Basic and Advanced Cardiac Life Support in Adults, Children, and Neonates With Suspected or Confirmed COVID-19. Visit **cpr.heart.org/covid** to see the most up-to-date guidance and algorithms.

 To find out about any updates or corrections to this text, visit **www.heart.org/courseupdates.**

Contents

Part 3
BLS for Adults

Contents

Appendix   93

Abbreviations

Abbreviation	Definition
AED	automated external defibrillator
AP	anteroposterior
BLS	Basic Life Support
CCF	chest compression fraction
CPR	cardiopulmonary resuscitation
ECG	electrocardiogram
ED	emergency department
EMS	emergency medical services
LUD	lateral uterine displacement
PAD	public access defibrillation
PPE	personal protective equipment
pVT	pulseless ventricular tachycardia
ROSC	return of spontaneous circulation
T-CPR	telecommunicator-assisted CPR

Contents

General Course Concepts

Welcome to the American Heart Association Basic Life Support (BLS) Provider Course. BLS is the foundation for saving lives after cardiac arrest. In this course, you will learn the skills of high-quality cardiopulmonary resuscitation (CPR) for victims of all ages. You will practice delivering these skills both as a single rescuer and as a member of a multirescuer team. The skills you learn in this course will enable you to

- Recognize cardiac arrest
- Activate the emergency response system early
- Respond quickly and confidently

Despite important advances in prevention, sudden cardiac arrest remains a leading cause of death in many countries. About half of cardiac arrests are unwitnessed. Outcome from out-of-hospital cardiac arrest remains poor. Only about 10% of adult patients with nontraumatic cardiac arrest who are treated by emergency medical services (EMS) survive to hospital discharge.

This course will help you give victims the best chance of survival.

BLS Course Objectives

The BLS Course focuses on what you need to know to perform high-quality CPR in a wide variety of settings. You will also learn how to respond to choking and other types of life-threatening emergencies.

After successfully completing the BLS Course, you should be able to

- Describe the importance of high-quality CPR and its impact on survival
- Describe all the steps in the Chains of Survival
- Apply the BLS concepts of the Chains of Survival
- Recognize the signs of someone needing CPR
- Perform high-quality CPR for an adult, a child, and an infant
- Describe the importance of early use of an automated external defibrillator (AED)
- Demonstrate the appropriate use of an AED
- Provide effective ventilation by using a barrier device
- Describe the importance of teams in multirescuer resuscitation
- Perform as an effective team member during multirescuer CPR
- Describe the technique for relief of foreign-body airway obstruction for an adult, a child, and an infant

Course Description

This course prepares you to perform high-quality CPR skills. CPR is a lifesaving procedure for a victim who has signs of cardiac arrest (ie, unresponsive, no normal breathing, and no pulse). The 2 key components of CPR are **chest compressions** and **breaths.**

High-quality CPR improves a victim's chances of survival. Study and practice the characteristics of high-quality CPR so that you can perform each skill effectively.

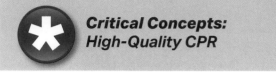

Critical Concepts: High-Quality CPR

- *Start compressions within 10 seconds after recognizing cardiac arrest.*
- *Push hard, push fast: Compress at a rate of 100 to 120/min with a depth of*
  - *At least 2 inches (5 cm) for adults but no more than 2.4 inches (6 cm)*
  - *At least one third the depth of the chest, approximately 2 inches (5 cm), for children*
  - *At least one third the depth of the chest, approximately 1½ inches (4 cm), for infants*
- *Allow complete chest recoil after each compression. Avoid leaning on the chest between compressions.*
- *Minimize interruptions in compressions (try to limit interruptions to less than 10 seconds).*
- *Give effective breaths. Deliver each breath over 1 second, enough to make the victim's chest rise. Avoid excessive ventilation.*

Completion Requirements

To successfully complete this course and receive your BLS course completion card, you must do the following:

- Participate in hands-on interactive demonstrations of high-quality CPR skills
- Pass the Adult CPR and AED Skills Test
- Pass the Infant CPR Skills Test
- Score at least 84% on the exam in the instructor-led course (or successfully complete the online portion of the HeartCode® BLS course)

Skills Tests

You must pass 2 skills tests to receive your BLS course completion card. During the course, you will have an opportunity to learn and practice chest compressions, bag-mask ventilation, and using an AED. After practice, your instructor will test your skills by reading a brief scenario. You will be asked to respond as you would in a real-life situation. The instructor will not coach or help you during the skills tests.

Exam

The exam is open resource. This means that you may refer to print or digital resources while you are taking the exam. You may not, however, discuss the exam questions with other students or your instructor. Examples of resources that you may use include notes you take in class, this Provider Manual, and the American Heart Association's *Handbook of Emergency Cardiovascular Care for Healthcare Providers*.

Your Approach to a Resuscitation Attempt

The BLS techniques and sequences you will learn offer 1 approach to a resuscitation attempt. But every situation is unique. Your response will be determined by

- Available emergency equipment
- Availability of trained rescuers
- Level of training expertise
- Local protocols

Personal Protective Equipment

Personal protective equipment (PPE) helps protect rescuers from health or safety risks. PPE will vary based on situations and protocols. It can include a combination of items, such as medical gloves, eye protection, gowns/full-body suits, high-visibility clothing, safety footwear, and safety helmets.

Ask your local health authority or regulatory body about the PPE protocols for your role.

The *BLS Provider Manual*

Read your *BLS Provider Manual* carefully. Study the skills and lifesaving sequences. During the course, you'll apply this knowledge as a rescuer in simulated emergency scenarios. Your BLS Provider Manual can serve as a resource long after you complete your course.

Age Definitions

In this course, age definitions are as follows:

- Infants: younger than 1 year of age (excluding newly born infants in the delivery room)
- Children: 1 year of age to puberty (signs of puberty are chest or underarm hair in males; any breast development in females)
- Adults: adolescents (ie, after the onset of puberty) and older

Callout Boxes

This manual includes Critical Concepts boxes that call attention to specific content.

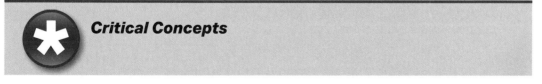

Critical Concepts

These boxes contain important information you must know, including specific risks associated with certain interventions and additional background on key topics.

Review Questions

Answer the review questions provided at the end of each Part. You may use these to confirm your understanding of important BLS concepts.

Part 2

The Chain of Survival

For many years, the American Heart Association has adopted, supported, and helped develop the concept of emergency cardiovascular care. The term *Chain of Survival* provides a useful metaphor for the elements of the emergency cardiovascular care systems-of-care concept. The Chain of Survival shows the actions that must take place to give the cardiac arrest victim the best chance of survival. Each link is independent, yet connected, to the links before and after. If any link is broken, the chance for a good outcome decreases.

Learning Objectives

At the end of this Part, you will be able to

- Describe the importance of high-quality CPR and its impact on survival
- Describe all of the steps in the Chain of Survival
- Apply the BLS concepts of the Chain of Survival

Overview

Cardiac arrest can happen anywhere—on the street, at home, or in a hospital emergency department (ED), inpatient bed, or intensive care unit. Elements in the system of care and order of actions in the Chain of Survival differ based on the situation. Care will depend on whether the victim has the arrest outside the hospital or inside the hospital. Care also depends on whether the victim is an adult, child, or infant.

Actions in the Chain of Survival differ according to setting (in-hospital vs out-of-hospital) and age group. Here are the specific Chains of Survival (Figure 1):

- Pediatric in-hospital cardiac arrest
- Pediatric out-of-hospital cardiac arrest
- Adult in-hospital cardiac arrest
- Adult out-of-hospital cardiac arrest

Figure 1. The American Heart Association 2020 Chains of Survival. Links in the Chain of Survival will differ based on whether the arrest occurs in or out of the hospital and the age of the victim. **A,** Pediatric In-Hospital Chain of Survival. **B,** Pediatric Out-of-Hospital Chain of Survival. **C,** Adult In-Hospital Chain of Survival. **D,** Adult Out-of-Hospital Chain of Survival.

A

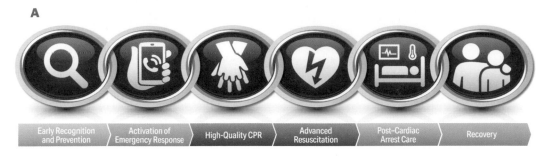

Early Recognition and Prevention | Activation of Emergency Response | High-Quality CPR | Advanced Resuscitation | Post–Cardiac Arrest Care | Recovery

B

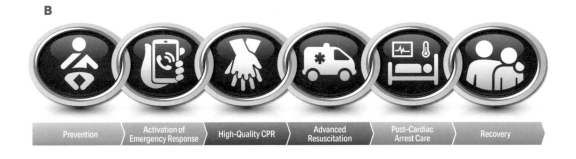

Prevention | Activation of Emergency Response | High-Quality CPR | Advanced Resuscitation | Post–Cardiac Arrest Care | Recovery

C

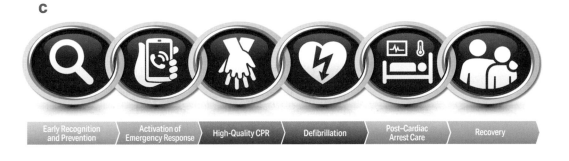

Early Recognition and Prevention | Activation of Emergency Response | High-Quality CPR | Defibrillation | Post–Cardiac Arrest Care | Recovery

D

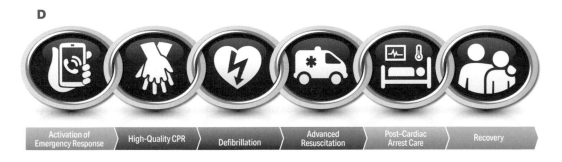

Activation of Emergency Response | High-Quality CPR | Defibrillation | Advanced Resuscitation | Post–Cardiac Arrest Care | Recovery

Chain of Survival Elements

Although there are slight differences in the Chains of Survival based on the age of the victim and the location of the cardiac arrest, each includes the following elements:

- Prevention and preparedness
- Activating the emergency response system
- High-quality CPR, including early defibrillation
- Advanced resuscitation interventions
- Post–cardiac arrest care
- Recovery

Prevention and Preparedness

Prevention and preparedness are the foundation of early recognition of cardiac arrest and rapid response.

Out-of-hospital. Most out-of-hospital adult cardiac arrests are unexpected and happen at home. Successful outcomes depend on early high-quality CPR and rapid defibrillation in the first few minutes after the arrest. Organized community programs that prepare the public to respond quickly to a cardiac arrest are critical to improving outcomes.

Prevention includes measures to improve the health of individuals and communities. *Preparedness* includes public awareness programs and training to help people recognize the signs of a heart attack and cardiac arrest and take effective action. Community CPR training and emergency response system development are important.

Emergency telecommunicators (ie, call takers, dispatchers) who give CPR instructions help increase rates of bystander CPR and improve outcomes. This telecommunicator-assisted CPR (T-CPR) enables the general public to perform high-quality CPR and early defibrillation.

Mobile phone apps or text messages can be used to summon members of the public who are trained in CPR. Mobile phone apps/mapping can help rescuers locate the nearest AED.

Widespread AED availability supports early defibrillation and saves lives. Public access defibrillation (PAD) programs are designed to reduce the time to defibrillation by placing AEDs in public places and training laypeople to use them.

In-hospital. In the hospital setting, *preparedness* includes early recognition and rapid response to the patient who may need resuscitation. For adult patients in the hospital, cardiac arrest usually happens as a result of serious respiratory or circulatory conditions that get worse. Healthcare providers can predict and prevent many of these arrests by careful observation, preventive care, and early treatment of prearrest conditions.

Once a provider recognizes cardiac arrest, immediate activation of the emergency response system, early high-quality CPR, and rapid defibrillation are essential. Many institutions conduct ongoing training in resuscitation response. Some maintain rapid response teams or medical emergency teams.

Activating the Emergency Response System

Out-of-hospital. Activating the emergency response system usually means shouting for nearby help and phoning 9-1-1 or the local emergency response number. In the workplace, every employee should know how to activate the emergency response system in their setting (Figure 2A). The sooner a rescuer activates the emergency response system, the sooner the next level of care will arrive.

In-hospital. Activation of the emergency response system in the hospital setting is specific to each institution (Figure 2B). A provider may activate a code, summon the rapid response team or medical emergency team, or ask someone else to do it. The sooner a provider activates the emergency response system, the sooner the next level of care will arrive.

Figure 2. Activate the emergency response system in your setting. **A,** Out-of-hospital setting in the workplace. **B,** In-hospital setting.

A

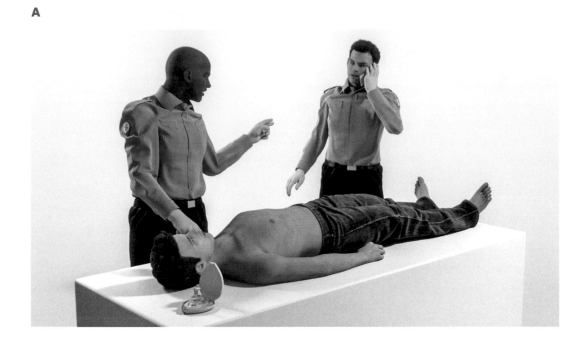

B

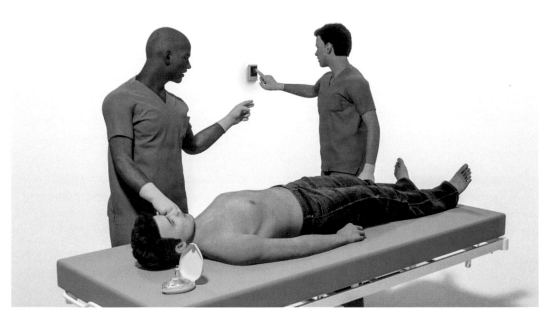

High-Quality CPR, Including Early Defibrillation

Out-of-hospital and in-hospital. High-quality CPR with minimal interruptions and early defibrillation are the actions most closely related to good resuscitation outcomes. High-quality CPR started immediately after cardiac arrest combined with early defibrillation can double or triple the chances of survival. These time-sensitive interventions can be provided both by members of the public and by healthcare providers. Bystanders who are not trained in CPR should at least provide chest compressions (also called *Hands-Only CPR*). Even without training, bystanders can perform chest compressions with guidance from emergency telecommunicators over the phone (T-CPR).

Advanced Resuscitation Interventions

Out-of-hospital and in-hospital. Advanced interventions may be performed by medically trained providers during a resuscitation attempt. Some advanced interventions are obtaining vascular access, giving medications, and placing an advanced airway. Others are obtaining a 12-lead electrocardiogram (ECG) or starting advanced cardiac monitoring. In both settings, high-quality CPR and defibrillation are key interventions that are the foundation of a successful outcome.

Out-of-hospital. Lay rescuers provide high-quality CPR and defibrillation with an AED until a multirescuer team takes over the resuscitation attempt. This high-performance team will continue high-quality CPR and defibrillation and may perform advanced interventions.

In-hospital. The high-performance team in a hospital may include physicians, nurses, respiratory therapists, pharmacists, and others. In addition to advanced interventions, extracorporeal CPR may be used in certain resuscitation situations.

Post–Cardiac Arrest Care

Out-of-hospital. After return of spontaneous circulation (ROSC), all cardiac arrest victims receive post–cardiac arrest care. Post–cardiac arrest care includes routine critical care support, such as artificial ventilation and blood pressure management. This care begins in the field and continues during transport to a medical facility.

In-hospital. A multidisciplinary team provides this advanced level of care. Providers focus on preventing the return of cardiac arrest and tailor specific therapies to improve long-term survival. Post–cardiac arrest care may occur in the ED, cardiac catheterization lab (cath lab), intensive care unit, or coronary care unit.

The patient may undergo a cardiac catheterization procedure. During this procedure, a catheter is inserted in an artery (most frequently the groin or wrist) and threaded through the blood vessels to the patient's heart to evaluate heart function and blood flow. Some cardiac problems, such as a blocked artery, may be fixed or other problems diagnosed.

Recovery

Recovery from cardiac arrest continues long after hospital discharge. Depending on the outcome, the survivor of cardiac arrest may need specific interventions. Interventions may be needed to address the underlying cause of cardiac arrest or to provide cardiac rehabilitation. Some patients need rehabilitation focused on neurological recovery. Psychological support for the patient and family are important during the recovery period. Rescuers also may benefit from psychological support.

Comparison of the In-Hospital and Out-of-Hospital Chains of Survival

Five key elements affect all Chains of Survival (Table 1). Those elements are initial support, resuscitation teams, available resources, resuscitation constraints, and level of complexity. Table 1 shows key differences in initial support, resuscitation teams, and available resources between the in-hospital and out-of-hospital settings. Resuscitation constraints and level of complexity are the same in both settings.

Table 1. Comparison of 5 Key Elements in the Chains of Survival

Element	In-hospital cardiac arrest	Out-of-hospital cardiac arrest
Initial support	Depends on an **in-hospital system** of appropriate **surveillance**, **monitoring**, and **prevention** with **responsive primary provider teams**	Depends on **community** and **EMS providers** for support
Resuscitation teams	Resuscitation efforts depend on • The smooth interaction of an institution's **various departments** and services (such as the patient ward, ED, cardiac cath lab, and intensive care unit) • **A multidisciplinary team of professional providers**, which includes physicians, nurses, respiratory therapists, pharmacists, counselors, and others	Resuscitation efforts depend on • **Lay rescuers** who need to recognize an unresponsive victim and quickly activate the emergency response system • **Lay rescuers** who perform CPR and use an AED (if available) until a high-performance team takes over resuscitation efforts • **EMS**, who transports the victim to a medical facility for continued care
Available resources	Depending on the facility, in-hospital **multidisciplinary teams** may have immediate access to additional personnel as well as resources of the **ED**, **cardiac cath lab**, and **intensive care unit**.	Available resources may be limited in the out-of-hospital settings: • **AED access:** AEDs may be available through a local **PAD program** or included in emergency or **first aid equipment**. • Untrained rescuers: **T-CPR** helps untrained rescuers perform high-quality CPR. • EMS high-performance teams: The **only resources may be those they brought with them.** Additional backup resources and equipment may take some time to arrive.
Resuscitation constraints	Factors that may affect both settings include **crowd control**, **family presence**, **space constraints**, **resources**, **training**, **patient transport**, and **device failures**.	
Level of complexity	Resuscitation attempts, both in and out of the hospital, are typically **complex**. They require teamwork and coordination between rescuers and care providers.	

Key Differences in Adult and Pediatric Chains of Survival

In adults, cardiac arrest is often sudden and frequently results from a cardiac cause. In children, however, cardiac arrest is often secondary to respiratory failure or shock. Both respiratory failure and shock can be life-threatening.

Prevention of cardiac arrest is the first link in the pediatric Chains of Survival (Figures 1A and B). Early identification of respiratory or circulatory problems and appropriate treatment may prevent progression to cardiac arrest. Early identification also may maximize survival.

Review Questions

1. In which locations do most out-of-hospital cardiac arrests occur?
   a. Healthcare clinics
   b. Homes
   c. Recreational facilities
   d. Shopping centers

2. Which is the most common cause of cardiac arrest in children?
   a. Cardiac problem
   b. Congenital or acquired heart defect
   c. Respiratory failure or shock
   d. Infection and sepsis

3. What is the third link in the adult out-of-hospital Chain of Survival?
   a. Advanced life support
   b. High-quality CPR
   c. Prevention
   d. Defibrillation

See Answers to Review Questions in the Appendix.

Part 3

BLS for Adults

This section describes BLS for adults. You will learn to perform high-quality CPR skills, both as a single rescuer and as a member of a multirescuer team.

Use adult BLS skills for victims who are adolescents (ie, after the onset of puberty) and older.

Learning Objectives

In this Part, you will learn to

- Recognize the signs of someone needing CPR
- Perform high-quality CPR for an adult
- Provide effective ventilation with a barrier device

Basic Framework for CPR

Anyone can be a lifesaving rescuer for a cardiac arrest victim (Figure 3). The particular CPR skills a rescuer uses depend on several variables, such as level of training, experience, and confidence (ie, rescuer proficiency). Other variables are the type of victim (child vs adult), available equipment, and other rescuers. A single rescuer with limited training or who has training but limited equipment can do Hands-Only CPR. A rescuer with more training can do 30:2 CPR. When several rescuers are present, they can perform multirescuer-coordinated CPR.

Here are some examples:

- **Hands-Only CPR.** A single rescuer with little training and no equipment who witnesses a cardiac arrest in a middle-aged man might provide only chest compressions until help arrives.
- **30:2 CPR.** A police officer trained in BLS who finds an adolescent in cardiac arrest will provide both chest compressions and breaths by using a ratio of 30 compressions to 2 breaths.
- **High-performance team.** Three emergency responders who are called to assist a woman in cardiac arrest will perform multirescuer-coordinated CPR: rescuer 1 performs chest compressions; rescuer 2 gives breaths with a bag-mask device; rescuer 3 uses the AED. Rescuer 3 also assumes the role of CPR Coach. A CPR Coach helps team members perform high-quality CPR and minimize pauses in chest compressions.

Figure 3. Building blocks of CPR.

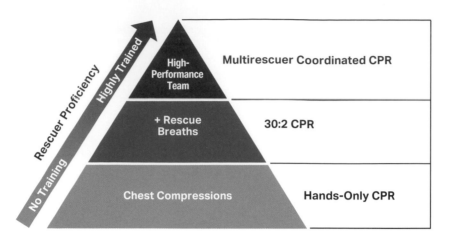

High-Performance Rescue Teams

Coordinated efforts by several rescuers during CPR may increase the chances for a successful resuscitation. High-performance teams divide tasks among team members during a resuscitation attempt.

As a team member, you will want to perform high-quality CPR skills to make your maximum contribution to each resuscitation team effort.

See Part 5 for more about team performance.

Main Components of CPR

The main components of CPR are

- Chest compressions
- Airway
- Breathing

You will learn about each of these throughout this course.

Adult BLS Algorithm for Healthcare Providers

The Adult BLS Algorithm for Healthcare Providers outlines steps for single rescuers and multiple rescuers of an unresponsive adult (Figure 4). Once you learn the skills presented in this Part, use this algorithm as a quick reference for providing high-quality CPR to an adult who is in cardiac arrest.

Figure 4. Adult BLS Algorithm for Healthcare Providers.

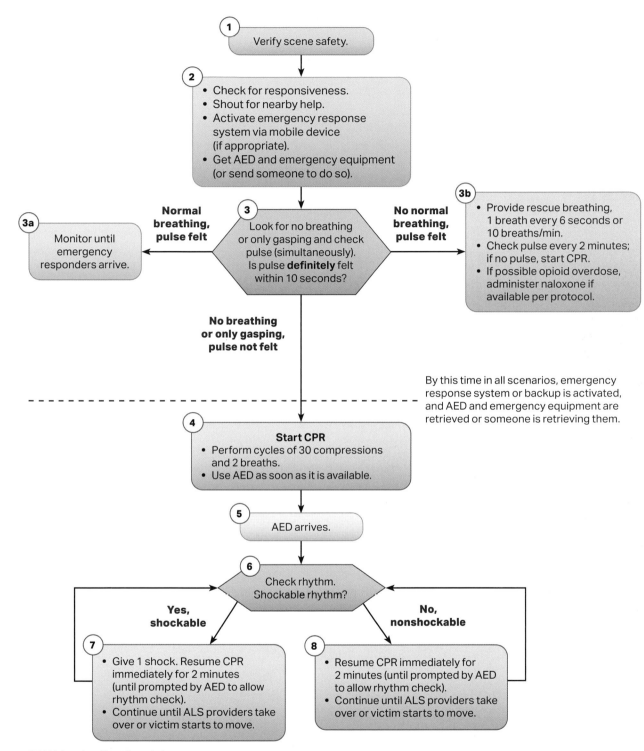

© 2020 American Heart Association

A rescuer who arrives at the side of a potential cardiac arrest victim should follow these sequential steps on the algorithm:

Step 1: Verify scene safety.

Make sure that the scene is safe for you and the victim.

Step 2: Check for responsiveness.

Tap the victim's shoulders. Shout, "Are you OK?" If the victim is not responsive, activate the emergency response system via mobile device. Get the AED or send someone to do so.

Step 3: Assess for breathing and a pulse.

Check for a pulse to determine next actions. To minimize delay in starting CPR, you should assess breathing and pulse at the same time. This should take no more than 10 seconds.

Steps 3a and 3b: Determine next actions based on whether breathing is normal and if a pulse is felt:

- **If the victim is breathing normally and a pulse is felt,** monitor the victim.
- **If the victim is not breathing normally but a pulse is felt:**
  - Provide rescue breathing at a rate of 1 breath every 6 seconds, or 10 breaths per minute.
  - Check for a pulse about every 2 minutes. Perform high-quality CPR if you do not feel a pulse.
  - If you suspect opioid use, give naloxone if available and follow your local protocols.
- **If the victim is not breathing normally or is only gasping and has no pulse,** begin high-quality CPR (Step 4).

Step 4: Start high-quality CPR, with 30 chest compressions followed by 2 breaths. Use an AED as soon as it is available.

Steps 5 and 6: Use the AED as soon as it is available. Follow the AED directions to check the rhythm.

Step 7: If the AED detects a shockable rhythm, give 1 shock. Resume CPR immediately until prompted by the AED to allow a rhythm check, about every 2 minutes. Continue CPR and using the AED until advanced life support providers take over or the victim begins to breathe, move, or otherwise react.

Step 8: If the AED detects a nonshockable rhythm, resume high-quality CPR until prompted by the AED to allow a rhythm check, about every 2 minutes. Continue CPR and using the AED until advanced life support providers take over or the victim begins to breathe, move, or otherwise react.

For a complete explanation of each step, see the Adult 1-Rescuer BLS Sequence in the Appendix.

High-Quality CPR Skills: Adults

Learning the skills in this section will prepare you to provide high-quality CPR to adults.

Assess for Breathing and a Pulse

Assess the victim for normal breathing and a pulse (Figure 5). This will help you determine the next appropriate actions.

To minimize delay in starting CPR, you should assess breathing at the same time as you check the pulse. This should take at least 5 seconds but no more than 10 seconds.

Breathing

To check for breathing, scan the victim's chest for rise and fall *for no more than 10 seconds.*

- **If the victim is breathing:** Monitor the victim until additional help arrives.
- **If the victim is not breathing or is only gasping:** Be prepared to begin high-quality CPR. Gasping is not normal breathing and is a sign of cardiac arrest.

Critical Concepts:
Agonal Gasps

Agonal gasps may be present in the first minutes after sudden cardiac arrest. Agonal gasps are not normal breathing.

A person who gasps usually appears to be drawing air in very quickly. The mouth may be open, and the jaw, head, or neck may move with gasps. Gasps may appear forceful or weak. Some time may pass between gasps because they usually happen at a slow, irregular rate. The gasp may sound like a snort, snore, or groan.

Gasping is not normal breathing. It is a sign of cardiac arrest.

Checking for the Carotid Pulse on an Adult

To perform a pulse check on an adult, feel for a carotid pulse (Figure 5).

If you do not definitely feel a pulse within 10 seconds, begin high-quality CPR, starting with chest compressions.

Figure 5. Check for breathing and a pulse at the same time.

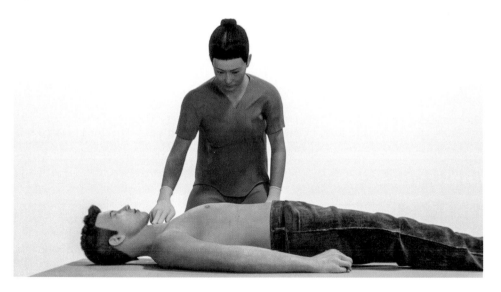

Follow these steps to find and feel for the carotid pulse:
- Locate the trachea (on the side closest to you), using 2 or 3 fingers (Figure 6A).
- Slide those fingers into the groove between the trachea and the muscles at the side of the neck, where you can feel the carotid pulse (Figure 6B).
- Feel for a pulse *for at least 5 but no more than 10 seconds*. If you do not definitely feel a pulse, begin CPR, starting with chest compressions.

Figure 6. Finding the carotid pulse. **A,** Locate the trachea. **B,** Gently feel for the carotid pulse.

A

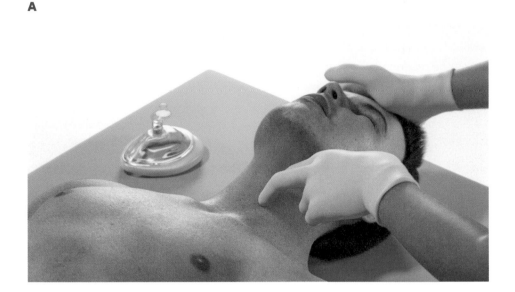

B

In all scenarios, by the time a breathing-and-pulse check indicates cardiac arrest, the following should already be happening:

- Someone has activated the emergency response system.
- Someone has gone to get the AED.

Perform High-Quality Chest Compressions

The foundation of CPR is high-quality chest compressions. Compressing the chest during CPR pumps blood from the heart to the brain and then to the rest of the body. Each time you stop chest compressions, the blood flow from the heart to the brain and other organs decreases significantly. Once you resume compressions, it takes several compressions to bring the blood flow back up to the levels present before the interruption. Thus, the more often you interrupt chest compressions and the longer the interruptions are, the lower the blood supply to the brain and critical organs.

When a victim is not breathing normally or is only gasping and has no pulse, begin CPR, starting with chest compressions.

Position Victim

Position the victim faceup on a firm, flat surface, such as the floor or a backboard. This will help ensure that the chest compressions are as effective as possible. If the victim is on a soft surface, such as a mattress, the force from the chest compressions will simply push the victim's body into the soft surface. A firm surface allows compression of the chest and the heart to create adequate blood flow.

Compression-to-Ventilation Ratio

Single rescuers should use the compression-to-ventilation ratio of 30 compressions to 2 breaths when giving CPR to victims of any age.

Compression Rate

Compress at a rate of 100 to 120/min. This rate is the same for compressions in all cardiac arrest victims.

Compression Depth

Compress the chest at least 2 inches (5 cm). As you practice this skill, remember that chest compressions are more often too shallow than too deep. However, it is possible to compress too deeply. Compressing the chest more than 2.4 inches (6 cm) in adults may decrease effectiveness of the compression and cause injuries. Using a CPR-quality feedback device can help you reach the optimal compression depth of 2 to 2.4 inches (5 to 6 cm).

Chest Recoil

Allow the chest to recoil (reexpand) completely after each compression. *Chest recoil* (reexpansion of the chest) allows blood to flow into the heart. Incomplete chest recoil reduces the filling of the heart between compressions and reduces the blood flow created by chest compressions. To help ensure complete recoil, avoid leaning on the chest between compressions. Chest compression and chest recoil times should be about equal.

Interruptions in Chest Compressions

Minimize interruptions in chest compressions. Shorter duration of interruptions in chest compressions is associated with better outcome. The proportion of time that rescuers perform chest compressions during CPR is called *chest compression fraction* (CCF). A CCF of at least 60% increases the likelihood of ROSC, shock success, and survival to hospital discharge. With good teamwork and training, rescuers can often achieve 80% or greater. This should be the goal in all team resuscitation events.

Do not move the victim while CPR is in progress unless the victim is in a dangerous environment (such as a burning building) or you believe you cannot perform CPR effectively under the current circumstances.

When help arrives, the resuscitation team, because of local protocol, may choose to continue CPR at the scene or transport the victim to an appropriate facility while continuing rescue efforts. High-quality BLS is key at all times during the resuscitation event.

Chest Compression Technique

Follow these steps to perform chest compressions on an adult:

1. Position yourself at the victim's side.
   a. Make sure the victim is lying faceup on a firm, flat surface. If the victim is facedown, carefully roll the person over. If you suspect a head or neck injury, try to keep the

head, neck, and torso in a line when rolling the victim to a faceup position. It is best if someone can assist you in rolling the victim.

2. Position your hands and body to perform chest compressions:

   a. Place the heel of one hand in the center of the victim's chest, on the lower half of the breastbone (sternum) (Figure 7A).

   b. Put the heel of your other hand on top of the first hand.

   c. Straighten your arms and position your shoulders directly over your hands.

3. Give chest compressions at a rate of 100 to 120/min.

4. Press down at least 2 inches (5 cm) with each compression; this requires hard work. For each chest compression, make sure you push straight down on the victim's breastbone (Figure 7B).

5. At the end of each compression, always allow the chest to recoil completely. Avoid leaning on the chest between compressions.

6. Minimize interruptions of chest compressions. (You will learn to combine compressions with ventilation next.)

Figure 7. A, Place the heel of your hand on the breastbone, in the center of the chest. **B,** Correct position of the rescuer during chest compressions.

A

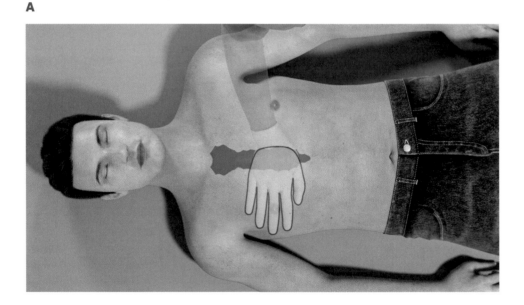

B

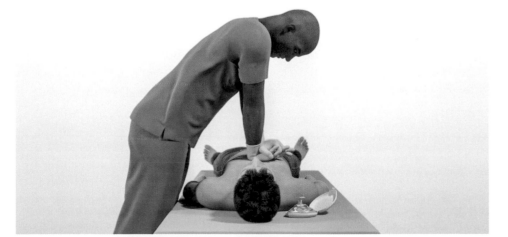

Alternate Technique for Chest Compressions

If you have difficulty pushing deeply during compressions, do the following:

- Put one hand on the breastbone to push on the chest.
- Grasp the wrist of that hand with your other hand to support the first hand as you push down on the chest (Figure 8).

This technique may be helpful for rescuers with joint conditions, such as arthritis.

Figure 8. Alternate technique for giving chest compressions to an adult.

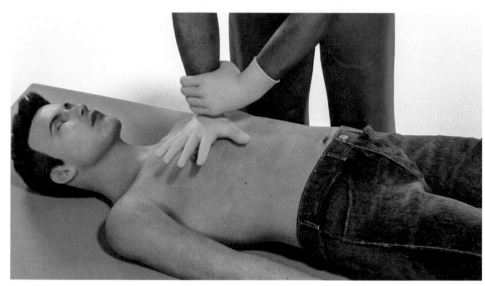

Compressions for a Pregnant Woman

Do not delay providing chest compressions for a pregnant woman in cardiac arrest. High-quality CPR, including respiratory support and early medical intervention, can increase the mother's and the infant's chance of survival. If you do not perform CPR on a pregnant woman when needed, the lives of both the mother and the infant are at risk. Perform high-quality chest compressions and ventilation for a pregnant woman just as you would for any victim of cardiac arrest. For more information, see Figure 44 and sequence in the Appendix.

Be aware that when a visibly pregnant woman (approximately 20 weeks) is lying flat on her back, the uterus compresses the large blood vessels in the abdomen. This pressure can interfere with blood flow to the heart generated by the chest compressions. Manual lateral uterine displacement (LUD) (ie, manually moving the uterus to the patient's left to relieve the pressure on the large blood vessels) can help relieve this pressure.

If additional rescuers are present and rescuers are trained, perform continuous LUD in addition to high-quality BLS (Figure 9). If the woman is revived, place her on her left side. This may help improve blood flow to her heart and, therefore, to the baby.

Figure 9. Manual LUD during CPR. **A,** 1-handed technique. **B,** 2-handed technique.

A   B

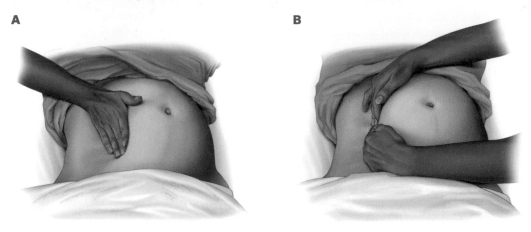

Critical Concepts:
Perform High-Quality Chest Compressions

- *Use a ratio of 30 compressions to 2 breaths.*
- *Compress at a rate of 100 to 120/min, with a depth of at least 2 inches (5 cm) for adults.*
- *Allow complete chest recoil after each compression. Do not lean on the chest between compressions.*
- *Minimize interruptions in chest compressions. Try to limit pauses in compressions to less than 10 seconds. The goal is a CCF of at least 60%; with good teamwork, rescuers can often achieve 80% or higher.*

Give Breaths

Opening the Airway

For breaths to be effective, the victim's airway must be open. Two methods for opening the airway are

- Head tilt–chin lift
- Jaw thrust

Important: If you suspect a head or neck injury, use the jaw-thrust maneuver to reduce neck and spine movement. If the jaw thrust does not open the airway, use the head tilt–chin lift maneuver.

When multiple rescuers are available, one rescuer can perform a jaw thrust while another rescuer provides breaths with a bag-mask device. The third rescuer will give chest compressions.

Head Tilt–Chin Lift

Follow these steps to perform a head tilt–chin lift (Figure 10):

1. Place one hand on the victim's forehead and push with your palm to tilt the head back.
2. Place the fingers of the other hand under the bony part of the lower jaw, near the chin.
3. Lift the jaw to bring the chin forward.

When performing a head tilt–chin lift, make certain that you

- Avoid pressing deeply into the soft tissue under the chin because this might block the airway
- Do not close the victim's mouth completely

Figure 10. The head tilt–chin lift maneuver. **A,** Obstruction by the tongue. When a victim is unresponsive, the tongue can block the upper airway. **B,** The head tilt–chin lift maneuver lifts the tongue, relieving the airway obstruction.

A　　　　　　　　　　　　　　　　　　　　**B**

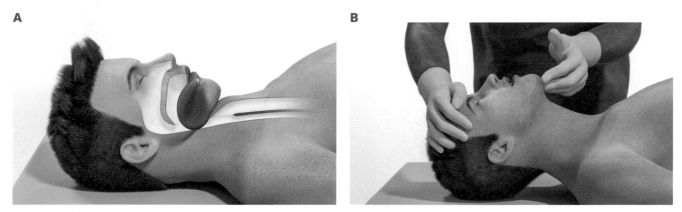

Jaw Thrust

When the head tilt–chin lift doesn't work or when you suspect a spinal injury, use the jaw-thrust maneuver (Figure 11).

Follow these steps to perform a jaw thrust:

1. Position yourself at the victim's head.
2. Place one hand on each side of the victim's head. You may rest your elbows on the surface where the victim is lying.
3. Place your fingers under the angle of the victim's lower jaw and lift with both hands, displacing the jaw forward (Figure 11).
4. If the victim's lips close, push the lower lip with your thumbs to open the lips.

If the jaw thrust does not open the airway, use a head tilt–chin lift.

Figure 11. Jaw thrust.

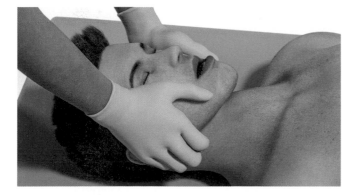

Barrier Devices for Giving Breaths

When giving breaths during CPR, standard precaution is to use a barrier device. Examples are pocket masks (preferred) and face shields. Rescuers should replace face shields with a pocket mask at the first opportunity.

Infection from CPR is extremely unlikely. Only a few cases have been reported. Yet, the US Occupational Safety and Health Administration requires that healthcare workers use standard precautions when performing CPR in the workplace.

Pocket Masks

For mouth-to-mask breaths, use a pocket mask (Figure 12). Pocket masks usually have a 1-way valve that diverts exhaled air, blood, or bodily fluids away from the rescuer. The 1-way valve allows the rescuer's breath to enter the victim's mouth and nose and diverts the victim's exhaled air away from the rescuer.

Pocket masks are available in different sizes for adults, children, and infants (Figure 12). Effective use of the pocket mask barrier device requires instruction and practice.

Figure 12. Adult, child, and infant pocket masks.

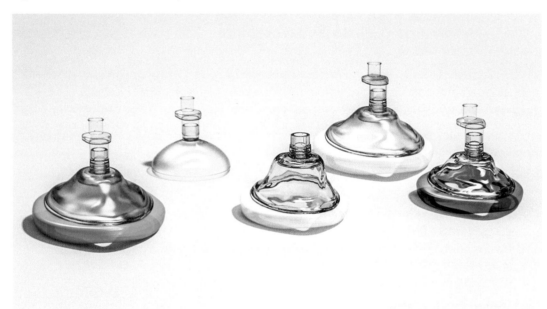

To use a pocket mask, position yourself at the victim's side. This position is ideal for 1-rescuer CPR because you can give breaths and perform chest compressions without repositioning yourself every time you change from compressions to giving breaths.

Follow these steps to open the airway with a head tilt–chin lift and give breaths with a pocket mask:

1. Position yourself at the victim's side.
2. Place the pocket mask on the victim's face, using the bridge of the nose as a guide for correct positioning.
3. Seal the pocket mask against the face.
   a. Using your hand that is closer to the top of the victim's head, place your index finger and thumb along the top edge of the mask.
   b. Place the thumb of your other hand along the bottom edge of the mask.
   c. Place the remaining fingers of your second hand along the bony margin of the jaw and lift the jaw. Perform a head tilt–chin lift to open the airway (Figure 10).
   d. While you lift the jaw, press firmly and completely around the outside edge of the mask to seal the pocket mask against the face (Figure 13).
4. Deliver each breath over 1 second, enough to make the victim's chest rise.

Figure 13. Press firmly and completely around the outside edge of the mask to seal the pocket mask against the face.

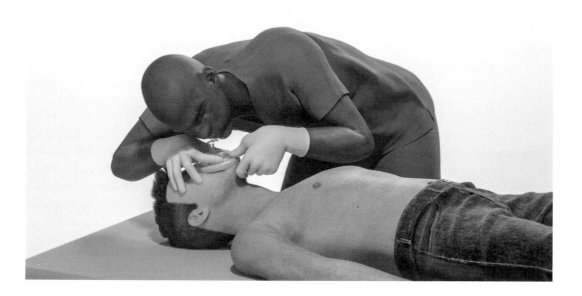

Critical Concepts:
Adult Breaths

Remember: When interrupting chest compressions to give 2 breaths with a barrier device, be sure that you

- Deliver each breath over 1 second
- Note visible chest rise with each breath
- Resume chest compressions in less than 10 seconds

Oxygen Content of Exhaled Air

The air we breathe in contains about 21% oxygen. The air we breathe out contains about 17% oxygen. This means that the air a rescuer breathes out still contains plenty of oxygen to provide the victim with much-needed oxygen.

Bag-Mask Devices

Use a bag-mask device, if available, (Figure 14) to provide positive-pressure ventilation to a victim who is either not breathing or not breathing normally. The device consists of a bag attached to a face mask. If the bag is self-inflating, you may use it with or without an oxygen supply. If not attached to oxygen flow, it provides about 21% oxygen from room air. Some bag-mask devices include a 1-way valve. The type of valve may vary from one device to another.

Face masks are available in a variety of sizes. Common sizes are infant (small), child (medium), and adult (large). For a proper fit, the mask should

- Extend from the bridge of the nose to just above the lower edge of the chin
- Cover the nose and mouth; make sure the mask does not apply pressure to the eyes (Figure 15)

The flexible, cushioned mask should provide an airtight seal. If the seal is not airtight, ventilation will be ineffective.

Bag-mask ventilation during CPR is more effective when 2 rescuers provide it together. One rescuer opens the airway and seals the mask against the face while the other squeezes the bag.

All BLS providers should be able to use a bag-mask device. Proficiency in this ventilation technique requires practice.

Figure 14. Bag-mask device.

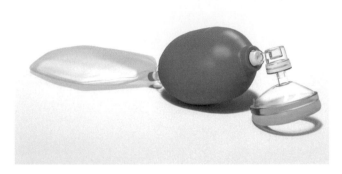

Figure 15. Proper area of the face for face mask application. Note that the mask should not apply pressure to the eyes.

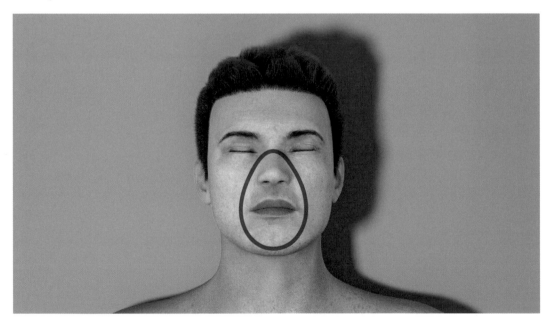

Bag-Mask Ventilation Technique (1 Rescuer)

To open the airway with a head tilt–chin lift and use a bag-mask device to give breaths to the victim, follow these steps:

1. Position yourself directly above the victim's head.
2. Place the mask on the victim's face, using the bridge of the nose as a guide for correct positioning. Use the E-C clamp technique to hold the mask in place while you lift the jaw to hold the airway open (Figure 16).
   a. Perform a head tilt.
   b. Place the mask on the face with the narrow portion at the bridge of the nose.

    c. Use the thumb and index finger of one hand to make a "C" on the side of the mask, pressing the edges of the mask to the face.

    d. Use the remaining fingers to lift the angles of the jaw (3 fingers form an "E"). Open the airway, and press the face to the mask.

  3. Squeeze the bag to give breaths while watching for chest rise. Deliver each breath over 1 second, with or without the use of supplemental oxygen.

Figure 16. E-C clamp technique of holding the mask while lifting the jaw. **A,** Side view. **B,** Aerial view.

A

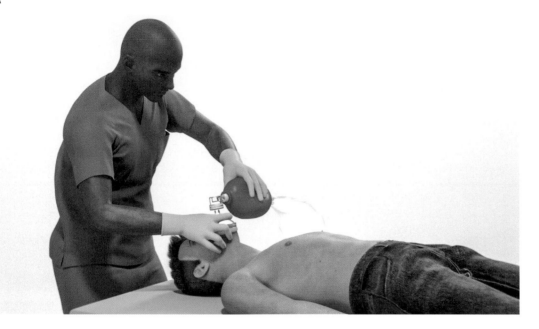

B

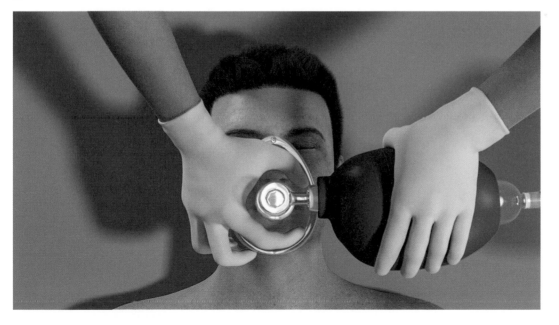

Bag-Mask Ventilation Technique (2 or More Rescuers)

When 3 or more rescuers are present, 2 of them working together can provide more effective and efficient bag-mask ventilation than 1 rescuer can. Two rescuers work together in this way (Figure 17):

1. Rescuer 1, positioned directly above the victim, opens the airway and positions the bag-mask device, following the steps described in the Bag-Mask Ventilation Technique (1 Rescuer) section.
   a. This rescuer should be careful not to press too hard on the mask, because doing so could push the patient's jaw down and block the airway.
2. Rescuer 2, positioned at the victim's side, squeezes the bag.

Figure 17. Two-rescuer bag-mask ventilation.

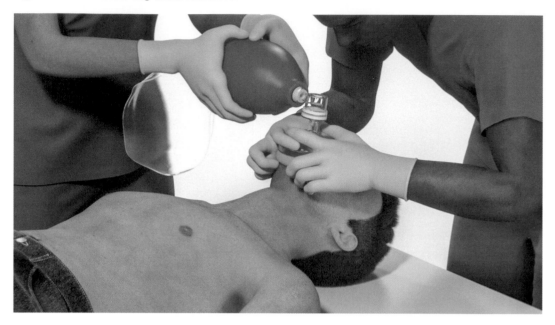

Ventilation for a Victim With a Stoma or Tracheostomy Tube

When ventilating a victim who has a stoma or tracheostomy tube, position the mask over the stoma or tube and use the previously described techniques. A pediatric mask may be more effective than an adult mask. If the chest doesn't rise, you may connect the bag-mask device directly to the tracheostomy tube. If the chest still does not rise, you may need to close the victim's mouth while providing breaths over the stoma or tracheostomy tube.

 Critical Concepts:
Two Rescuers for Jaw Thrust and Bag-Mask Ventilation

During CPR, jaw thrust and bag-mask ventilation are more efficiently performed when 2 or more rescuers are providing ventilation. One rescuer must be positioned above the victim's head and use both hands to open the airway, lift the jaw, and hold the mask to the face while the second rescuer squeezes the bag. The second rescuer is positioned at the victim's side.

Adult 2-Rescuer BLS

When you encounter an unresponsive adult and other rescuers are available, work together to follow the steps outlined in the Adult BLS Algorithm for Healthcare Providers (Figure 4). When more rescuers are available for a resuscitation attempt, more tasks can be performed at the same time.

The first rescuer who arrives at the side of a potential cardiac arrest victim should quickly assess the scene for safety and check the victim for responsiveness. This rescuer should send another rescuer to activate the emergency response system and get the AED. As more rescuers arrive, assign tasks. Additional rescuers can help with bag-mask ventilation, compressions, and using the AED (Figure 18).

For complete step-by-step instructions on following the Adult BLS Algorithm for Healthcare Providers as part of a multirescuer team, see the Adult 2-Rescuer BLS Sequence in the Appendix.

Figure 18. Multiple rescuers can perform simultaneous tasks during a resuscitation attempt.

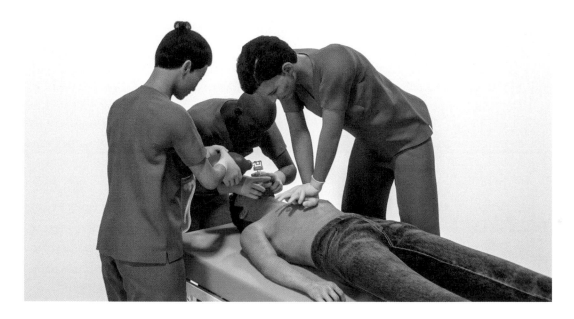

Team Roles and Duties for 2 or More Rescuers

When more rescuers are available for a resuscitation attempt, they can perform more tasks at the same time. In two-rescuer CPR (Figure 19), each rescuer has specific tasks.

Rescuer 1: Provide Compressions

Position yourself at the victim's side.

- Make sure the victim is faceup on a firm, flat surface.
- Perform chest compressions.
  - Compress at a rate of 100 to 120/min.
  - Compress the chest at least 2 inches (5 cm) for adults.
  - Allow the chest to recoil completely after each compression; avoid leaning on the victim's chest between compressions.
  - Minimize interruptions in compressions (try to limit any interruptions in chest compressions to less than 10 seconds).
  - Use a compression-to-ventilation ratio of 30:2.
  - Count compressions out loud.
- Switch compressors about every 5 cycles or every 2 minutes (more frequently if fatigued). Take less than 5 seconds to switch.

Rescuer 2: Provide Breaths

Position yourself at the victim's head.

- Maintain an open airway by using either
  - Head tilt–chin lift or
  - Jaw thrust
- Give breaths, watching for chest rise and avoiding excessive ventilation.
- Encourage the first rescuer to
  - Perform compressions that are deep enough and fast enough
  - Allow complete chest recoil between compressions
- When only 2 rescuers are available, switch with the compressor about every 5 cycles or every 2 minutes, taking less than 5 seconds to switch.

Figure 19. Two-rescuer CPR.

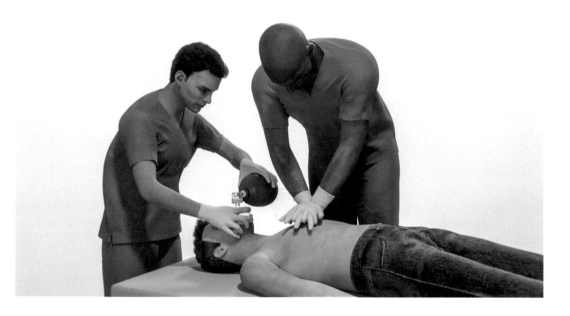

 Critical Concepts: High-Performance Teams

- *When giving compressions, rescuers should switch compressors after every 5 cycles of CPR (about every 2 minutes), or sooner if fatigued.*
- *As additional rescuers arrive, they can help with bag-mask ventilation, compressions, and using the AED and other emergency equipment (Figure 18).*

Effective Team Performance to Minimize Interruptions in Compressions

Effective teams communicate continuously. If the Compressor counts out loud, the rescuer providing breaths can anticipate when to give breaths. This will help the rescuer prepare to give breaths efficiently and minimize interruptions in compressions. Also, the count will alert both rescuers when the time for a switch is approaching.

Delivering effective chest compressions is hard work. If the Compressor tires, chest compressions will not be as effective. To reduce rescuer fatigue, switch Compressors about every 5 cycles (or every 2 minutes) or sooner if needed. To minimize interruptions, switch roles when the AED is analyzing the rhythm. Take less than 5 seconds to switch.

Some BLS providers have special training in coaching CPR to help the resuscitation team minimize interruptions in chest compressions. This role is called the *CPR Coach*.

What Is a CPR Coach?

Many resuscitation teams now include the role of CPR Coach. The CPR Coach supports performance of high-quality BLS skills, allowing the Team Leader to focus on other aspects of clinical care. Studies have shown that resuscitation teams with a CPR Coach perform higher-quality CPR with higher CCF and shorter pause durations than teams that do not use a CPR Coach.

The CPR Coach does not need to be a separate role; it can be most effectively blended into the current responsibilities of the Monitor/Defibrillator. The CPR Coach's main responsibilities are to help team members provide high-quality CPR and minimize pauses in compressions. The CPR Coach needs a direct line of sight to the Compressor, so they should stand next to the defibrillator. Here is a description of the CPR Coach's actions:

Coordinate the start of CPR: As soon as a patient is identified as having no pulse, the CPR Coach says, "I am the CPR Coach," and tells rescuers to begin chest compressions. The CPR Coach can adjust the environment to help ensure high-quality CPR. They can lower the bedrails or the bed, get a step stool, or roll the victim to place a backboard and defibrillator pads to better facilitate high-quality CPR.

Coach to improve the quality of chest compressions: The CPR Coach gives feedback about performance of compression depth, rate, and chest recoil. They state the CPR feedback device's data to help the Compressor improve performance. This is useful because visual assessment of CPR quality is often inaccurate.

State the midrange targets: The CPR Coach states the specific midrange targets so that compressions and ventilation are within the recommended range. For example, they should tell the Compressor to compress at a rate of 110 per minute instead of a rate between 100 and 120 per minute.

Coach to the midrange targets: The CPR Coach gives team members feedback about their ventilation rate and volume. If needed, they also remind the team about compression-to-ventilation ratio.

Help minimize the length of pauses in compressions: The CPR Coach communicates with the team to help minimize the length of pauses in compressions. Pauses happen when the team defibrillates, switches Compressors, and places an advanced airway.

Review Questions

Scenario: A 53-year-old man collapses and becomes unresponsive. You witness his collapse and are the first rescuer at the scene, where the man is lying motionless on the floor.

1. Which is the first action you should take in this situation?
   a. Activate the emergency response system.
   b. Start high-quality CPR, beginning with chest compressions.
   c. Start providing rescue breaths.
   d. Verify that the scene is safe for you and the victim.

2. The man doesn't respond when you tap his shoulders and shout, "Are you OK?" What is your best next action?

 a. Check his pulse.

 b. Start high-quality CPR.

 c. Start providing rescue breaths.

 d. Shout for nearby help.

3. Several rescuers respond, and you ask them to activate the emergency response system and retrieve the AED. As you check for a pulse and breathing, you notice that the man is gasping for air and making snorting sounds. You do not feel a pulse. What is your best next action?

 a. Start high-quality CPR, beginning with chest compressions.

 b. Monitor the victim until additional, more experienced help arrives.

 c. Provide rescue breathing by delivering 1 breath every 6 seconds.

 d. Find someone to help by retrieving the nearest AED.

4. What is the ratio of chest compressions to breaths when providing CPR to an adult?

 a. 10 compressions to 2 breaths

 b. 15 compressions to 2 breaths

 c. 30 compressions to 2 breaths

 d. 100 compressions to 2 breaths

5. What are the rate and depth for chest compressions on an adult?

 a. A rate of 60 to 80 compressions per minute and a depth of approximately 1 inch

 b. A rate of 80 to 100 compressions per minute and a depth of approximately 1½ inches

 c. A rate of 120 to 140 compressions per minute and a depth of approximately 2½ inches

 d. A rate of 100 to 120 compressions per minute and a depth of at least 2 inches

6. What action should you take when more rescuers arrive?

 a. Assign tasks to other rescuers and rotate compressors every 2 minutes or more frequently if needed to avoid fatigue.

 b. Continue CPR while the AED is attached, even if you are fatigued.

 c. Wait for the most experienced rescuer to provide direction to the team.

 d. Direct the team to assign a Team Leader and roles while you continue CPR.

7. If you suspect that an unresponsive victim has head or neck trauma, what is the preferred method for opening the airway?

 a. Head tilt–chin lift

 b. Jaw thrust

 c. Head tilt–neck lift

 d. Avoid opening the airway

8. What is CCF?

 a. The force you use to compress the chest

 b. Compression-to-ventilation ratio

 c. Proportion of time that rescuers perform chest compressions during CPR

 d. Another term for *chest recoil*

See Answers to Review Questions in the Appendix.

Automated External Defibrillator for Adults and Children 8 Years of Age and Older

An *automated external defibrillator*, or AED, is a lightweight, portable, computerized device that can identify an abnormal heart rhythm that needs a shock. The AED can then deliver a shock that can stop the abnormal rhythm and allow the heart's normal rhythm to return. AEDs are simple to operate. They allow laypersons and healthcare providers to attempt defibrillation safely.

Learning Objectives

In this Part, you will learn about

- The importance of using an AED as soon as possible for adults and children 8 years of age and older
- The appropriate use of an AED for adults and children 8 years of age and older

Defibrillation

The AED identifies abnormal heart rhythms as shockable or nonshockable. Shockable rhythms are treated with defibrillation. *Defibrillation* is the medical term for interrupting or stopping an abnormal heart rhythm by using controlled electrical shocks. The shock stops the abnormal rhythm. This resets the heart's electrical system so a normal (organized) heart rhythm can return.

If effective circulation returns, the victim's heart muscle is once again able to pump blood. The victim will have a heartbeat that produces a palpable pulse (a pulse that can be felt by the rescuer). This is called *return of spontaneous circulation*, or ROSC. Signs of ROSC include breathing, coughing, or movement and a palpable pulse or measurable blood pressure.

Early Defibrillation

Early defibrillation increases the chance of survival from cardiac arrest that is caused by an abnormal or irregular heart rhythm, or an *arrhythmia*. Arrhythmias occur when the electrical impulses that cause the heart to beat happen too quickly, too slowly, or erratically. Two life-threatening shockable arrhythmias that cause cardiac arrest are pulseless ventricular tachycardia (pVT) and ventricular fibrillation.

- **pVT:** When the lower chambers of the heart (ventricles) begin contracting at a very fast pace, a rapid heart rate known as *ventricular tachycardia* develops. In extremely severe cases, the ventricles pump so quickly and inefficiently that there is no detectable pulse (ie, the "pulseless" in pVT). Body tissues and organs, especially the heart and brain, no longer receive oxygen.

- **Ventricular fibrillation:** In this arrest rhythm, the heart's electrical activity becomes chaotic. The heart muscles quiver in a fast, unsynchronized way so that the heart does not pump blood.

Early defibrillation, high-quality CPR, and all components of the Chain of Survival are necessary to improve chances of survival from pVT and ventricular fibrillation.

Public Access Defibrillation Programs

To provide early defibrillation, rescuers need to have an AED immediately available. Public access defibrillation (PAD) programs increase AED availability and train laypeople how to use them. PAD programs place AEDs in public places where large numbers of people gather, such as office buildings, airports, convention centers, and schools. They also place AEDs in communities where people are at higher risk for cardiac arrest, such as office buildings, casinos, and apartment buildings. Some PAD programs coordinate with local EMS so that telecommunicators can direct callers to the nearest AED.

Critical Concepts:
Maintaining the AED and Supplies

AEDs should be properly maintained according to the manufacturer's instructions. Someone should be designated to do the following:

- *Maintain the battery.*
- *Order and replace supplies, including AED pads (adult and pediatric).*
- *Replace used equipment,* including barrier devices (eg, pocket masks), gloves, razors (for shaving hairy chests), and scissors.*

*These items are sometimes kept in a separate emergency or first aid kit.

AED Arrival

Once the AED arrives, place it at the victim's side, near the rescuer who will operate it. This position provides ready access to AED controls and helps ensure easy placement of AED pads. It also allows a second rescuer to continue high-quality CPR from the opposite side of the victim without interfering with AED operation. Ensure that AED pads are placed directly on the skin and are not placed over clothing, medication patches, or implanted devices.

Using the AED

Know Your AED

AED equipment varies according to the model and manufacturer. But all AEDs operate in basically the same way. The universal steps for operating an AED can guide you in most situations. However, you should still be familiar with the AED used in your setting. For example, it is important to know whether you must manually power on your AED or whether it powers on automatically when you open the lid.

Operating an AED: Universal Steps

Begin by opening the AED. If needed, power it on. During a resuscitation attempt, follow the AED's prompts. These may be electronic voice prompts or digital screen prompts.

To reduce the time to shock delivery, try to perform the following 2 steps within 30 seconds after the AED arrives at the victim's side:

1. **Open** the carrying case (if applicable). **Power on the AED** (Figure 20) if needed.
    a. Some devices power on automatically when you open the lid or case.
    b. Follow the AED prompts.
2. **Attach the AED pads** to the victim's bare chest. Avoid placing the pads over clothing, medication patches, or implanted devices. Choose adult pads for victims 8 years of age and older. This should be done while a second rescuer continues CPR.
    a. Peel the backing away from the AED pads.
    b. Attach the adhesive AED pads to the victim's bare chest. Follow the placement diagrams on the pad (Figure 21). See Critical Concepts: AED Pad Placement Options later in Part 4 for common placement options.
    c. Attach the AED connecting cables to the AED device (some AEDs have preconnected cables).
3. "Clear" the victim and allow the AED to analyze the rhythm (Figure 22).
    a. When the AED prompts you, clear the victim during analysis. Be sure no one is touching the victim, not even the rescuer in charge of giving breaths.
    b. Some AEDs will tell you to push a button to allow the AED to begin analyzing the heart rhythm; others will analyze automatically. The AED may take a few seconds to analyze.
    c. The AED then tells you if the victim needs a shock.
4. If the AED advises a shock, it will tell you to **clear** the victim (Figure 23A) and then deliver a shock.
    a. Before delivering the shock, clear the victim. Do this by making sure that no one is touching the victim.
      - Loudly state a "clear the victim" message, such as "Everybody clear."
      - Look to be sure that no one is in contact with the victim.
    b. Press the Shock button (Figure 23B). The shock will produce a sudden contraction of the victim's muscles.
5. If the AED prompts that no shock is advised or after any shock is delivered, immediately resume CPR, starting with chest compressions (Figure 24).
6. After about 5 cycles or 2 minutes of CPR, the AED will prompt you to repeat Steps 3 and 4.

Figure 20. Power on the AED.

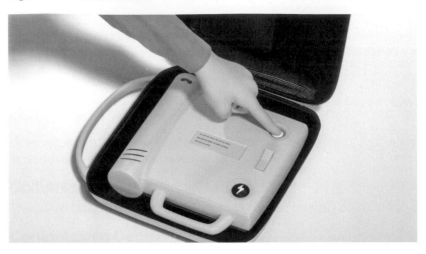

Figure 21. The AED operator attaches AED pads to the victim and then attaches the electrodes to the AED.

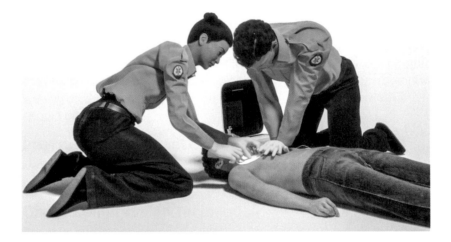

Figure 22. The AED operator clears the victim before rhythm analysis. If needed, the AED operator then activates the analyze feature of the AED.

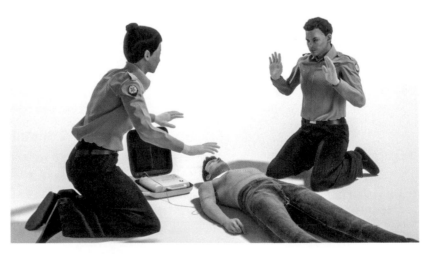

Figure 23. A, The AED operator clears the victim before delivering a shock. **B,** When everyone is clear of the victim, the AED operator presses the Shock button.

A

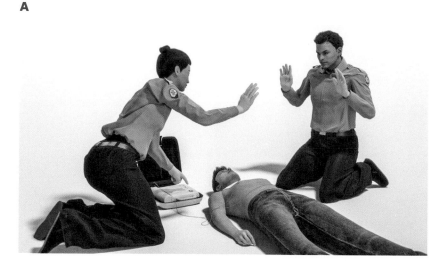

B

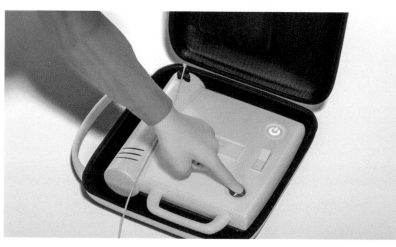

Minimize Time Between Last Compression and Shock Delivery

Research has shown that the shorter the time between the last compression and shock delivery, the better the chances of ROSC. Minimizing interruptions requires practice and team coordination, especially between the compressor and the AED operator.

Do Not Delay High-Quality CPR After AED Use

Immediately resume high-quality CPR, starting with chest compressions (Figure 24) after either of the following:

- The AED operator delivers a shock
- The AED prompts, "No shock advised"

After about 5 cycles or 2 minutes of high-quality CPR, the AED will prompt you to repeat Steps 3 and 4. Continue until advanced life support providers take over or the victim begins to breathe, move, or otherwise react.

Figure 24. If no shock is indicated and immediately after any shock delivered, rescuers start CPR, beginning with chest compressions.

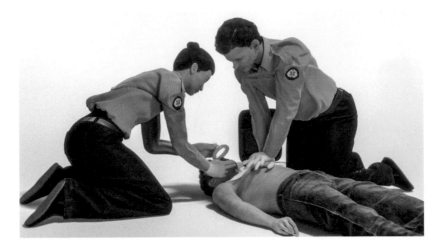

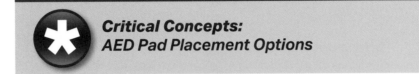

Critical Concepts:
AED Pad Placement Options

Place AED pads by following the diagram on the pads. The 2 common placements are anterolateral and anteroposterior (AP).

Anterolateral Placement

- *As shown in Figure 25A, place both pads on the victim's bare chest.*
- *Place one AED pad directly below the right collarbone.*
- *Place the other pad to the side of the left nipple, with the top edge of the pad a few inches below the armpit.*

AP Placement

- *As shown in Figure 25B, place one pad in the center of the victim's bare chest (anterior) and the other pad in the center of the victim's back (posterior).*

Or

- *Place one AED pad on the left side of the chest, between the left side of the victim's breastbone and left nipple. Place the other pad on the left side of the victim's back, next to the spine.*

Always place pads directly on the skin and avoid contact with clothing, medication patches, and implanted devices.

Figure 25. AED pad placement options on a victim. **A,** Anterolateral. **B,** Anteroposterior.

A

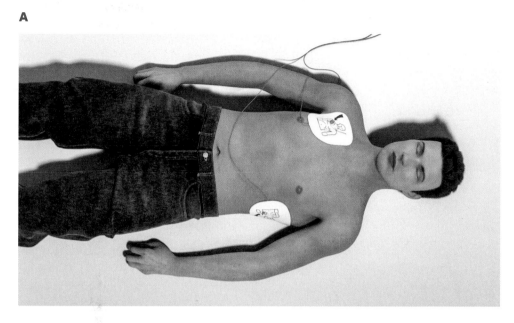

B

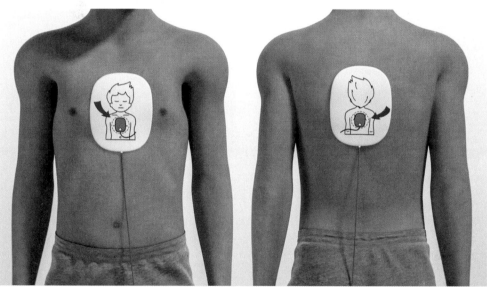

Child AED Pads

Your AED may include smaller pads designed specifically for children younger than 8 years of age. Do not use the child pads for an adult. Child pads deliver a shock dose that is too low for an adult and will likely not be successful. It is better to provide high-quality CPR than to attempt to shock an adult victim with child pads.

Special Circumstances

When placing AED pads, you may need to take additional actions when the victim

- Has a hairy chest
- Is immersed in water or has water or liquid covering the chest
- Has an implanted defibrillator or pacemaker
- Has a transdermal medication patch or other object on the surface of the skin where you need to place the AED pads
- Is a pregnant woman
- Is wearing jewelry or bulky clothing

Hairy Chest

The AED pads may stick to the chest hair and not to the skin on the chest. If this occurs, the AED will not be able to analyze the victim's heart rhythm and will display a "check electrodes" or "check electrode pads" message.

Remember to note whether the victim has a hairy chest *before you apply the pads*. Then, if needed, use the razor from the AED carrying case to shave the area where you will place the pads.

If you do not have a razor but do have a second set of pads, use the first set to remove the hair. Apply the first set of pads, press them down so they stick as much as possible, and quickly pull them off. Then apply the new second set of pads.

Presence of Water or Other Liquids

Water and other liquids conduct electricity. Do not use an AED in water.

- If the victim is in water, pull the victim out of the water.
- If the chest is covered with water or sweat, quickly wipe the chest before attaching the AED pads.
- If the victim is lying on snow or in a small puddle, you may use the AED after quickly wiping the chest.

Implanted Defibrillators and Pacemakers

Victims with a high risk for sudden cardiac arrest may have implanted defibrillators or pacemakers that automatically deliver shocks directly to the heart. If you place an AED pad directly over an implanted medical device, the implanted device may interfere with the delivery of the shock.

These devices are easy to identify because they create a hard lump beneath the skin that is most often in the left upper chest but can also be found in the right upper chest or abdomen. The lump can range from the size of a silver dollar to half the size of a deck of playing cards.

If you identify an implanted defibrillator/pacemaker:

- If possible, avoid placing the AED pad directly over the implanted device.
- Follow the normal steps for operating an AED.

Transdermal Medication Patches

Do not place AED pads directly on top of a medication patch. The patch may interfere with the transfer of energy from the AED pad to the heart. This could also cause small burns to the skin. Examples of medication patches are nitroglycerin, nicotine, pain medication, and hormone replacement therapy patches.

If it will not delay shock delivery, remove the patch, and wipe the area before attaching the AED pad.

To avoid the transfer of medication from the patch to you, wear protective gloves or use another type of barrier when removing the patch. Remember to avoid delays as much as possible.

Pregnant Woman

You should use an AED for a pregnant woman in cardiac arrest as you would for any cardiac arrest victim. Shock from the AED will not harm the baby. Without lifesaving treatment to the mother, the baby will not likely survive. If the woman is revived, place her on her left side. This helps improve blood flow to her heart and, therefore, to the baby.

Clothing and Jewelry

Quickly move bulky clothes out of the way. If a person's clothes are difficult to remove, you can still provide compressions over clothing. If an AED becomes available, remove all clothes that cover the chest because pads must not be placed over clothing. You do not need to remove a person's jewelry as long as it does not come into contact with the AED pads.

Review Questions

1. What is the most appropriate first step to take as soon as the AED arrives at the victim's side?
   a. Press the Analyze button.
   b. Apply the pads.
   c. Power on the AED.
   d. Press the Shock button.

2. Which step is one of the universal steps for operating an AED?
   a. Shaving the victim's hairy chest
   b. Placing the pads on the victim's bare chest
   c. Removing the victim from water
   d. Finding the victim's implanted pacemaker

3. If a victim of cardiac arrest has an implanted pacemaker or defibrillator, what special steps should you take?
   a. Avoid placing the AED pad directly over the implanted device.
   b. Avoid using the AED to prevent damage to the implanted device.
   c. Turn off the implanted device before applying the AED pads.
   d. Consider using pediatric pads to decrease the shock dose delivered.

4. What action should you take while the AED is analyzing the heart rhythm?
   a. Check the pulse.
   b. Continue chest compressions.
   c. Give rescue breaths only.
   d. Stand clear of the victim.

See Answers to Review Questions in the Appendix.

Team Dynamics

As a BLS provider, you may be involved in a multirescuer resuscitation attempt. Effective team dynamics increase the chances of a successful resuscitation. Everyone on the team must understand not just *what* to do in a resuscitation attempt but *how* to communicate and perform effectively as part of a multirescuer team.

Learning Objectives

At the end of this Part, you will be able to
- Describe the importance of teams in multirescuer resuscitation
- Perform as an effective team member during multirescuer CPR

Elements of Effective Team Dynamics

A successful resuscitation attempt depends on high-quality resuscitation skills, good communication, and effective team dynamics. All rescuers on the team must be able to respond rapidly and effectively in an emergency situation. Effective multirescuer team dynamics help give victims the best chance of survival.

Team dynamics during a resuscitation attempt include 3 elements:
- Roles and responsibilities
- Communication
- Debriefing

Roles and Responsibilities

Because every second matters during a resuscitation attempt, it is important to define clear roles and responsibilities as soon as possible.

Assign Roles and Responsibilities

When all team members know their jobs and responsibilities, the team functions more smoothly. Rescuers should clearly define roles as soon as possible and delegate tasks according to each team member's skill level. As soon as the victim is identified as *pulseless*, the CPR Coach will identify themselves and prompt the Compressor to begin chest compressions.

Figure 26 shows an example of a team formation with assigned roles.

Figure 26. Team diagram, including both BLS and advanced provider roles.

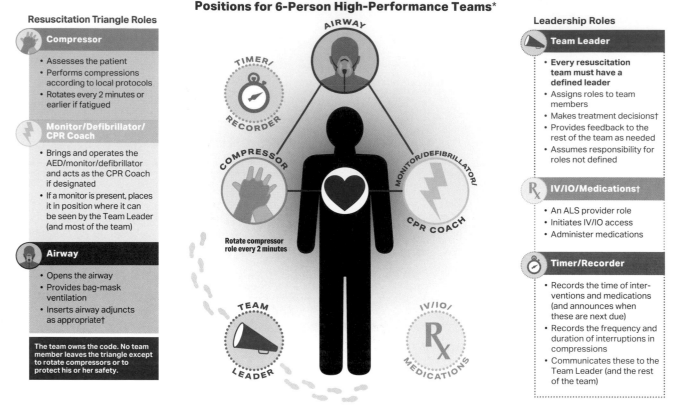

Positions for 6-Person High-Performance Teams*

Resuscitation Triangle Roles

Compressor
- Assesses the patient
- Performs compressions according to local protocols
- Rotates every 2 minutes or earlier if fatigued

Monitor/Defibrillator/ CPR Coach
- Brings and operates the AED/monitor/defibrillator and acts as the CPR Coach if designated
- If a monitor is present, places it in position where it can be seen by the Team Leader (and most of the team)

Airway
- Opens the airway
- Provides bag-mask ventilation
- Inserts airway adjuncts as appropriate†

The team owns the code. No team member leaves the triangle except to rotate compressors or to protect his or her safety.

Leadership Roles

Team Leader
- **Every resuscitation team must have a defined leader**
- Assigns roles to team members
- Makes treatment decisions†
- Provides feedback to the rest of the team as needed
- Assumes responsibility for roles not defined

IV/IO/Medications†
- An ALS provider role
- Initiates IV/IO access
- Administer medications

Timer/Recorder
- Records the time of interventions and medications (and announces when these are next due)
- Records the frequency and duration of interruptions in compressions
- Communicates these to the Team Leader (and the rest of the team)

Rotate compressor role every 2 minutes

*This is a suggested team formation. Roles may be adapted to local protocol.
†Roles and tasks are performed by advanced providers.

Know Your Limitations

All team members should know their limitations. The Team Leader needs to be aware of them as well. For example, advanced life support providers may be able to perform tasks that BLS providers would not be permitted to do. Some of these tasks are administering medications and performing intubation. Each team member should ask for assistance and advice early, before a situation starts to get worse.

Offer Constructive Intervention

Whether you are a team member or the Team Leader, there may be times when you need to point out another team member's incorrect or inappropriate actions. When this happens, it is important to intervene in a tactful and constructive way. This is especially important if someone is about to make a mistake on a drug, a dose, or an intervention.

Anyone on the team should speak up to stop someone else from making a mistake, regardless of role.

Communication

Share Knowledge

Knowledge sharing is important for effective team performance. Not only can it help ensure that everyone fully understands the situation, but it can also help the team treat patients more efficiently and effectively. Team Leaders should frequently ask for observations and feedback. This includes asking for good ideas about managing a resuscitation attempt as well as for observations about possible oversights.

Summarize and Reevaluate

Summarizing information aloud is helpful during a resuscitation attempt because it

- Provides an ongoing record of treatment
- Is a way to reevaluate the victim's status, the interventions, and the team's progress within the algorithm of care
- Helps team members respond to the victim's changing condition

Use Closed-Loop Communication

Closed-loop communication is an important technique used to prevent misunderstandings and treatment errors. It consists of the sender giving the message, the receiver repeating it back, and the sender then confirming it was heard correctly. To practice closed-loop communication, the Team Leader and team members should do the following:

Team Leader

- Call each team member by name and make eye contact when giving an instruction.
- Do not assign additional tasks until you are sure the team member understands the instruction.

Team members

- Confirm that you understand each task the Team Leader assigns to you by verbally acknowledging that task.
- Tell the Team Leader when you have finished a task.

Give Clear Messages

To help prevent misunderstandings and keep everyone focused, all team members should

- Use clear, concise language
- Speak loudly enough to be heard
- Speak in a tone that's both calm and confident

Show Mutual Respect

All team members should display mutual respect and a professional attitude, regardless of each rescuer's skill level or training. Emotions can run high during a resuscitation attempt. It's especially important for the Team Leader to speak in a friendly, controlled voice and avoid shouting or aggression.

Coaching and Debriefing

Coaching and debriefing are important in every resuscitation attempt. During the event, the CPR Coach will help improve performance of compressions and ventilation by ongoing coaching. They also will work with the Team Leader to minimize pauses in compressions during defibrillation and placement of an advanced airway.

After the resuscitation event, debriefing is an opportunity for the team to discuss how the resuscitation went, identify why the team took certain actions, and discuss whether anything can be improved in future events. Debriefing can occur immediately with the entire team or be scheduled at a later time with the team and others. It is an opportunity for education, quality improvement, and processing of emotions after participation in a stressful event.

Debriefing has been shown to

- Help individual team members perform better
- Aid in identifying system strengths and deficiencies

Implementing debriefing programs may improve patient survival after cardiac arrest.

Review Questions

1. After performing high-quality CPR for 5 minutes, the Team Leader frequently interrupts chest compressions to check for a pulse. Which action demonstrates constructive intervention?

   a. Ask another rescuer what he thinks should be done.

   b. Say nothing that contradicts the Team Leader.

   c. Suggest resuming chest compressions without delay.

   d. Wait until the debriefing session afterward to discuss it.

2. The Team Leader asks you to perform bag-mask ventilation during a resuscitation attempt, but you have not perfected that skill. What would be an appropriate action to acknowledge your limitations?

   a. Pick up the bag-mask device and give it to another team member.

   b. Pretend you did not hear the request and hope the Team Leader chooses someone else to do it.

   c. Tell the Team Leader you are not comfortable performing that task.

   d. Try to do it as best you can and hope another team member will see you struggling and take over.

3. What is the appropriate action to demonstrate closed-loop communication when the Team Leader assigns you a task?

   a. Repeat back to the Team Leader the task assigned to you.

   b. Nod your head as an acknowledgment of the assigned task.

   c. Start performing the assigned tasks, but do not speak, to minimize noise.

   d. Wait for the Team Leader to address you by name before you acknowledge the task.

See Answers to Review Questions in the Appendix.

BLS for Infants and Children

This section describes BLS for infants and children. In this course, *infants* are younger than 1 year of age (excluding the newly born), and *children* range from 1 year of age to puberty.

Learning Objectives

In this Part, you will learn to
- Perform high-quality CPR for a child
- Perform high-quality CPR for an infant

Pediatric BLS Algorithm for Healthcare Providers— Single Rescuer

The Pediatric BLS Algorithm for Healthcare Providers—Single Rescuer outlines the steps for a single rescuer of an unresponsive infant or child (Figure 27). Once you learn the skills presented in this Part, use the algorithm as a quick reference.

Figure 27. Pediatric BLS Algorithm for Healthcare Providers—Single Rescuer.

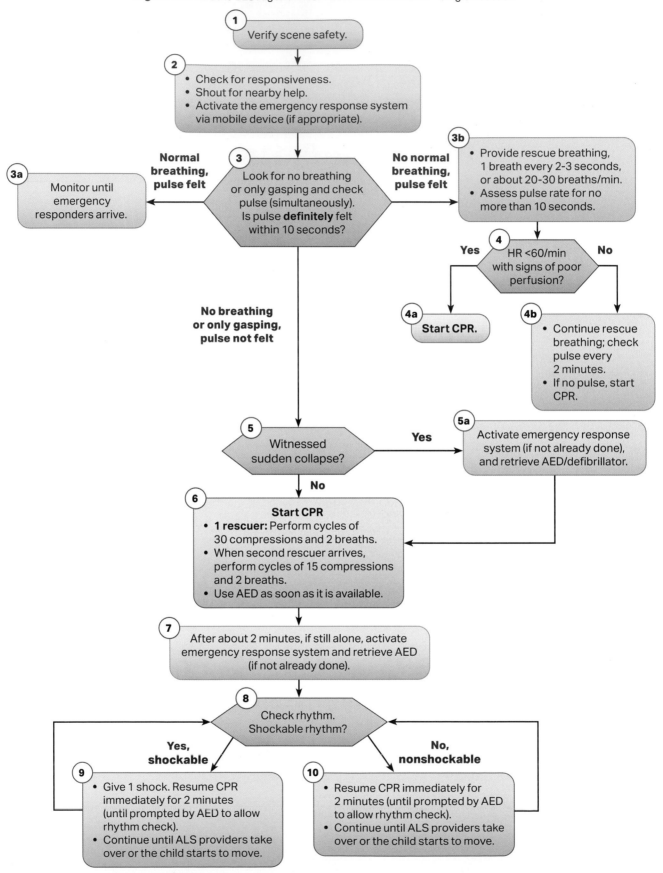

The first rescuer who arrives at the side of an infant or child who may be in cardiac arrest should follow these sequential steps on the algorithm:

Step 1: Verify scene safety.

Make sure the scene is safe for you and the victim.

Step 2: Check for responsiveness and get help.

Tap the child's shoulders. Shout, "Are you OK?" If the victim is not responsive, shout for help and activate the emergency response system via mobile device if appropriate.

Step 3: Assess for breathing and a pulse. Check for a pulse to determine next actions. To minimize delay in starting CPR, you should assess breathing and pulse at the same time. This should take no more than 10 seconds.

Steps 3a and 3b: Determine next actions based on whether breathing is normal and if a pulse is felt:

- **If the victim is breathing normally and a pulse is felt:**
  - Activate the emergency response system (if not already done).
  - Monitor the victim until emergency responders arrive.
- **If the victim is not breathing normally but a pulse is felt:**
  - Provide rescue breathing, with 1 breath every 2 to 3 seconds, or 20 to 30 breaths per minute.
  - Assess the pulse rate for 10 seconds.

Steps 4, 4a, and 4b: Is the heart rate less than 60/min with signs of poor perfusion?

- If yes, start CPR.
- If no, continue rescue breathing. Check for a pulse about every 2 minutes. If no pulse, start CPR.

Steps 5 and 5a: Was the sudden collapse witnessed?

If yes, activate the emergency response system (if not already done), and get the AED.

Step 6: If the collapse wasn't witnessed:

Start CPR with cycles of 30 compressions and 2 breaths. Use an AED as soon as it is available.

Step 7: After about 2 minutes, if you are still alone, activate the emergency response system and get an AED if not already done.

Step 8: Use the AED as soon as it is available.

Follow the AED directions to check the rhythm.

Step 9: If the AED detects a shockable rhythm, give 1 shock. Resume CPR immediately until prompted by the AED to allow a rhythm check, about every 2 minutes. Continue CPR and using the AED until advanced life support providers take over or the victim begins to breathe, move, or otherwise react.

Step 10: If the AED detects a nonshockable rhythm, resume high-quality CPR until prompted by the AED to allow a rhythm check, about every 2 minutes. Continue CPR and using the AED until advanced life support providers take over or the victim begins to breathe, move, or otherwise react.

For a complete explanation of each step, see the Infant and Child 1-Rescuer BLS Sequence in the Appendix.

High-Quality CPR Skills: Infants and Children

Mastering all the skills outlined in this section will prepare you to provide high-quality CPR to an unresponsive infant or child.

Assess for Breathing and a Pulse

Checking the infant or child for normal breathing and a pulse will help you determine the next appropriate actions. You should assess breathing and pulse at the same time. Take no more than 10 seconds to check both so that you can start CPR quickly, if necessary.

Breathing

To check for breathing, scan the victim's chest for rise and fall for *no more than 10 seconds*.

- **If the victim is breathing:** Monitor the victim until additional help arrives.
- **If the victim is not breathing or is only gasping:** The victim has respiratory arrest or (if no detectable pulse) cardiac arrest. (Gasping is not normal breathing and is a sign of cardiac arrest. See Critical Concepts: Agonal Gasps in Part 3.)

Pulse

Infant: To perform a pulse check in an infant, feel for a brachial pulse (Figure 28A). Here is how to check the brachial artery pulse:

1. Place 2 or 3 fingers on the inside of the upper arm, midway between the infant's elbow and shoulder.
2. Press your fingers down and attempt to feel the pulse for *at least 5 but no more than 10 seconds*.

Child: To perform a pulse check in a child, feel for a carotid or femoral pulse (Figure 28B and Figure 28C). Check the carotid pulse for a child by using the same technique as for an adult (see Part 3). Here is how to check the femoral artery pulse:

1. Place 2 or 3 fingers in the inner thigh, midway between the hip bone and the pubic bone and just below the crease where the leg meets the torso.
2. Feel for a pulse for at least 5 but no more than 10 seconds.

It can be difficult for BLS providers to determine the presence or absence of a pulse in any victim, particularly in an infant or child. If you do not *definitely feel a pulse within 10 seconds*, start high-quality CPR, beginning with chest compressions.

Figure 28. Pulse check. **A,** In an infant, feel for a brachial pulse. **B,** In a child, feel for a carotid pulse, or **C,** a femoral pulse.

A

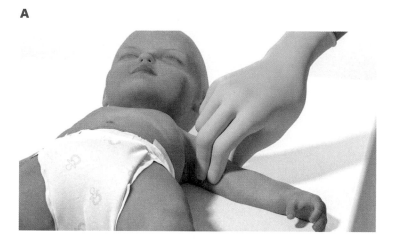

B

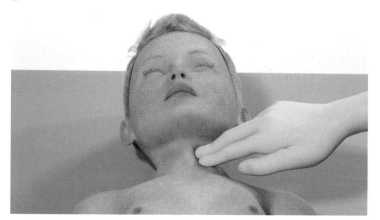

C

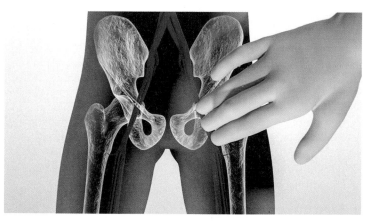

Signs of Poor Perfusion

Perfusion is the flow of oxygenated blood from the heart through the arteries to the body's tissues. To identify signs of poor perfusion, assess the following:

- **Temperature:** Cool extremities
- **Altered mental state:** Continued decline in consciousness/responsiveness
- **Pulses:** Weak pulses
- **Skin:** Paleness, mottling (patchy appearance), and, later, cyanosis (blue lips or skin)

Perform High-Quality Chest Compressions

High-quality chest compressions are the foundation of CPR. Perform compressions as described here to give an infant or child victim of cardiac arrest the best chance of survival.

Compression-to-Ventilation Ratio

The compression-to-ventilation ratio for single rescuers is the same in adults, children, and infants: **30:2**.

However, when 2 rescuers are attempting to resuscitate an infant or child, they should use a compression-to-ventilation ratio of **15:2**.

Compression Rate

The universal rate for compressions in all cardiac arrest victims is 100 to 120/min.

Compression Depth

For an infant, compress at least one third the AP diameter of the infant's chest (approximately 1½ inches, or 4 cm). For a child, compress at least one third the AP diameter of the chest (approximately 2 inches, or 5 cm) with each compression.

Chest Recoil

During CPR, chest recoil (reexpansion of the chest) allows blood to flow into the heart. Incomplete chest recoil reduces the filling of the heart between compressions and reduces the blood flow that chest compressions create. To help ensure complete recoil, avoid leaning on the chest between compressions. Chest compression and chest recoil times should be about equal.

Interruptions in Chest Compressions

Minimize interruptions in chest compressions. Shorter duration of interruptions in chest compressions is associated with better outcomes.

Chest Compression Techniques

For child chest compressions, use 1 or 2 hands. For most children, the compression technique is the same as for an adult: 2 hands (heel of one hand with heel of other hand on top of the first hand). For a small child, 1-handed compressions may be adequate to achieve the desired compression depth. Whether you use one hand or both hands, compress at least one third the AP diameter of the chest (approximately 2 inches, or 5 cm) with each compression.

For infants, single rescuers can use either the 2-finger or 2 thumb–encircling hands technique. If multiple rescuers are present, the 2 thumb–encircling hands technique is preferred. If you cannot compress the necessary depth on an infant with your fingers, you can use the heel of one hand. These techniques are described below.

Infant: 2-Finger Technique

Follow these steps to give chest compressions to an infant by using the 2-finger technique:

1. Place the infant on a firm, flat surface.
2. Place 2 fingers in the center of the infant's chest, just below the nipple line, on the lower half of the breastbone. Do not press the tip of the breastbone (Figure 29).
3. Give compressions at a rate of 100 to 120/min.
4. Compress at least one third the AP diameter of the infant's chest (approximately 1½ inches, or 4 cm).
5. At the end of each compression, make sure you allow the chest to completely recoil (reexpand); do not lean on the chest. Chest compression and chest recoil times should be about equal. Minimize interruptions in compressions (eg, to give breaths) to less than 10 seconds.

6. After every 30 compressions, open the airway with a head tilt–chin lift and give 2 breaths, each over 1 second. The chest should rise with each breath.

7. After about 5 cycles or 2 minutes of CPR, if you are alone and no one has activated the emergency response system, leave the infant (or carry the infant with you) and activate the emergency response system and get the AED.

8. Continue compressions and breaths at a ratio of 30 compressions to 2 breaths. Use the AED as soon as it is available. Continue until advanced life support providers take over or the infant begins to breathe, move, or otherwise react.

Figure 29. Two-finger chest compression technique for an infant.

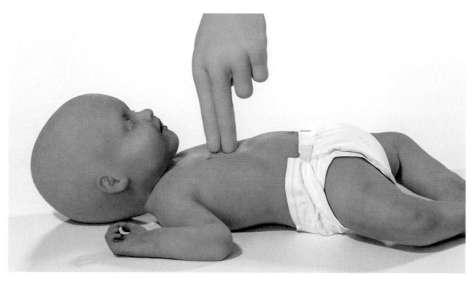

Infant: 2 Thumb–Encircling Hands Technique

The 2 thumb–encircling hands technique is the preferred technique when 2 rescuers provide CPR, but it can be used by 1 rescuer as well. This technique

- Produces better blood supply to the heart muscle
- Helps ensure consistent depth and force of chest compressions
- May generate higher blood pressures

Follow these steps to give chest compressions to an infant by using the 2 thumb–encircling hands technique:

1. Place the infant on a firm, flat surface.

2. Place both thumbs side by side in the center of the infant's chest, on the lower half of the breastbone. Your thumbs may overlap on very small infants. With the fingers of both hands, encircle the infant's chest and support the infant's back.

3. With your hands encircling the chest, use both thumbs to depress the breastbone (Figure 30) at a rate of 100 to 120/min.

4. Compress at least one third the AP diameter of the infant's chest (approximately 1½ inches, or 4 cm).

5. After each compression, release all pressure on the breastbone and allow the chest to recoil completely.

6. After every 15 compressions, pause briefly for the second rescuer to open the airway with a head tilt–chin lift and give 2 breaths, each over 1 second. The chest should rise with each breath. Minimize interruptions in compressions (eg, to give breaths) to less than 10 seconds.

7. Continue compressions and breaths at a ratio of 15 compressions to 2 breaths (for 2 rescuers). The rescuer providing chest compressions should switch roles with another provider about every 2 minutes to avoid fatigue so that chest compressions remain effective. Continue CPR until the AED arrives, advanced life support providers take over, or the infant begins to breathe, move, or otherwise respond.

An additional alternative for compressions on an infant or child is to use the heel of one hand. This technique may be useful for larger infants or if the rescuer has difficulty compressing to the appropriate depth with their fingers or thumbs.

Figure 30. Two thumb–encircling hands technique for an infant (2 rescuers).

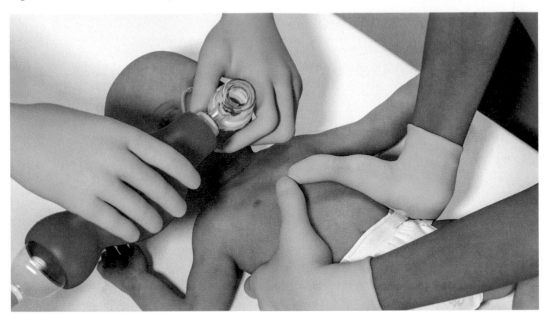

 Critical Concepts:
Compression Depth in Infants and Children vs Adults and Adolescents

- *Infants: At least one third the AP diameter of the chest, or approximately 1½ inches (4 cm)*
- *Children: At least one third the AP diameter of the chest, or approximately 2 inches (5 cm)*
- *Adults and adolescents: At least 2 inches, or 5 cm*

Give Breaths

Breaths Are Important for Infants and Children in Cardiac Arrest

When cardiac arrest occurs suddenly, the blood's oxygen content is typically adequate to meet the body's oxygen demands for the first few minutes after the arrest. Thus, for witnessed *sudden* cardiac arrest, chest compressions alone can be an effective way of distributing oxygen to the heart and brain.

However, cardiac arrest in infants and children may not be sudden and is often caused by respiratory complications. Infants and children who develop cardiac arrest often have respiratory failure or shock that reduces the oxygen content in the blood even before cardiac arrest occurs. As a result, for most infants and children in cardiac arrest, giving chest compressions alone does not deliver oxygenated blood to the heart and brain as effectively as giving both compressions and breaths. *Thus, it is vitally important that infants and children receive both compressions and breaths during high-quality CPR.*

Opening the Airway

As discussed in Opening the Airway in Part 3, for rescue breaths to be effective, the airway must be open. Two methods for opening the airway are the head tilt–chin lift and the jaw-thrust maneuver.

As with adults, if you suspect a neck injury, use the jaw-thrust maneuver. If the jaw thrust does not open the airway, use the head tilt–chin lift.

Critical Concepts:
Keep Infant's Head in the Neutral Position

If you tilt (extend) an infant's head beyond the neutral (sniffing) position, the infant's airway may become blocked. Maximize an open airway by positioning the infant with the neck in a neutral position so that the external ear canal is level with the top of the infant's shoulder.

Ventilation With a Barrier Device

Use a barrier device (eg, a pocket mask or face shield) or a bag-mask device for delivering breaths to an infant or child. See Barrier Devices for Giving Breaths and Bag-Mask Devices in Part 3 for detailed instructions.

When providing bag-mask ventilation for an infant or child, do the following:

1. Select a bag and mask of appropriate size. The mask must cover the victim's mouth and nose completely without covering the eyes or extending below the bottom edge of the chin.
2. Perform a head tilt–chin lift to open the victim's airway. Press the mask to the face as you lift the jaw, making a seal between the child's face and the mask.
3. Connect to supplemental oxygen when available.

Pediatric BLS Algorithm for Healthcare Providers—2 or More Rescuers

The Pediatric BLS Algorithm for Healthcare Providers—2 or More Rescuers outlines steps for a multirescuer team assisting an unresponsive infant or child (Figure 31).

Figure 31. Pediatric BLS Algorithm for Healthcare Providers—2 or More Rescuers.

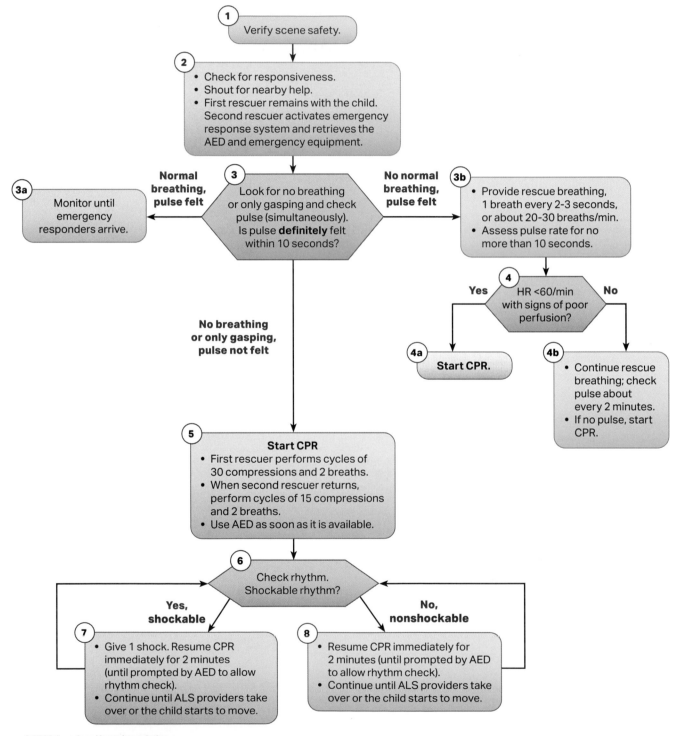

Infant and Child 2-Rescuer BLS

The first rescuer who arrives at the side of an unresponsive infant or child should quickly perform the first 2 steps on the algorithm. As more rescuers arrive, assign roles and responsibilities. As a multirescuer team, follow the algorithm's sequential steps. When more rescuers are available for a resuscitation attempt, they can perform some tasks at the same time.

Step 1: Verify scene safety.

Make sure that the scene is safe for you and the victim.

Step 2: Check for responsiveness and get help.

Tap the child's shoulders. Shout, "Are you OK?" If the victim is not responsive, shout for help and activate the emergency response via mobile device if appropriate. The first rescuer remains with the victim while the second rescuer activates the emergency response system and retrieves the AED and emergency equipment.

Step 3: Assess for breathing and a pulse.

Check for a pulse to determine next actions. To minimize delay in starting CPR, you should assess breathing and pulse at the same time. This should take no more than 10 seconds.

Steps 3a and 3b: Determine next actions based on whether breathing is normal and if a pulse is felt:

- **If the victim is breathing normally and a pulse is felt,** activate the emergency response system. Monitor the victim until emergency responders arrive.
- **If the victim is not breathing normally but a pulse is felt:**
  - Provide rescue breathing, with 1 breath every 2 to 3 seconds, or 20 to 30 breaths per minute.
  - Assess the pulse rate for 10 seconds.

Steps 4, 4a, and 4b: Is the heart rate less than 60/min (less than 6 beats in 10 seconds) with signs of poor perfusion?

- If yes, start CPR.
- If no, continue rescue breathing. Check for a pulse about every 2 minutes. If no pulse, start CPR.

Step 5: The first rescuer starts cycles of CPR with 30 compressions and 2 breaths. When the second rescuer returns, continue cycles of CPR with 15 compressions and 2 breaths. Use the AED as soon as it is available.

Step 6: Follow the AED directions to check the rhythm.

Step 7: If the AED detects a shockable rhythm, give 1 shock. Resume CPR immediately until prompted by the AED to allow a rhythm check, about every 2 minutes. Continue CPR and using the AED until advanced life support providers take over or the victim begins to breathe, move, or otherwise react.

Step 8: If the AED detects a nonshockable rhythm, resume high-quality CPR until prompted by the AED to allow a rhythm check, about every 2 minutes. Continue CPR and using the AED until advanced providers take over or the victim begins to breathe, move, or otherwise react.

For a complete explanation of each step, see Infant and Child 2-Rescuer BLS Sequence in the Appendix.

Review Questions

1. What is the correct compression-to-ventilation ratio for a single rescuer of a 3-year-old child?

   a. 15 compressions to 1 breath

   b. 15 compressions to 2 breaths

   c. 20 compressions to 2 breaths

   d. 30 compressions to 2 breaths

2. What is the correct compression-to-ventilation ratio for a 7-year-old child when 2 or more rescuers are present?

   a. 15 compressions to 1 breath

   b. 15 compressions to 2 breaths

   c. 20 compressions to 2 breaths

   d. 30 compressions to 2 breaths

3. For what age victim is the 2 thumb–encircling hands technique recommended?

   a. A child younger than 3 years of age

   b. A child older than 3 years of age

   c. An infant older than 1 year

   d. An infant younger than 1 year

4. What is the correct chest compression depth for a child?

   a. At least one fourth the depth of the chest, or approximately 1 inch (2.5 cm)

   b. At least one third the depth of the chest, or approximately 1½ inches (4 cm)

   c. At least one third the depth of the chest, or approximately 2 inches (5 cm)

   d. At least one half the depth of the chest, or approximately 3 inches (7.6 cm)

5. What is the correct chest compression depth for an infant?

   a. At least one fourth the depth of the chest, or approximately 1 inch (2.5 cm)

   b. At least one third the depth of the chest, or approximately 1½ inches (4 cm)

   c. At least one third the depth of the chest, or approximately 2 inches (5 cm)

   d. At least one half the depth of the chest, or approximately 2½ inches (6.4 cm)

See Answers to Review Questions in the Appendix.

Automated External Defibrillator for Infants and Children Younger Than 8 Years of Age

Rescuers may use an AED when attempting to resuscitate infants and children younger than 8 years of age. This Part will help you understand how to use an AED for victims in this age range.

Learning Objectives

In this Part, you will learn

- The importance of using an AED as early as possible for infants and children younger than 8 years of age
- How to use an AED for infants and children younger than 8 years of age

Know Your AED

Although all AEDs operate in basically the same way, AED equipment varies according to model and manufacturer. You should be familiar with the AED used in your setting.

See Operating an AED: Universal Steps in Part 4.

Pediatric-Capable AEDs for Reduced Shock Doses

Most AED models are designed for both pediatric and adult resuscitation attempts. These AEDs deliver a reduced shock dose when pediatric pads are used.

One common way to reduce a shock dose is by attaching a pediatric dose attenuator to the AED (Figure 32). An attenuator reduces the shock dose by about two thirds. Typically, an attenuator delivers the reduced shock via child pads. A pediatric dose attenuator frequently comes preconnected to the pediatric pads.

Figure 32. A pediatric dose attenuator reduces the shock dose an AED delivers. This attenuator uses child pads.

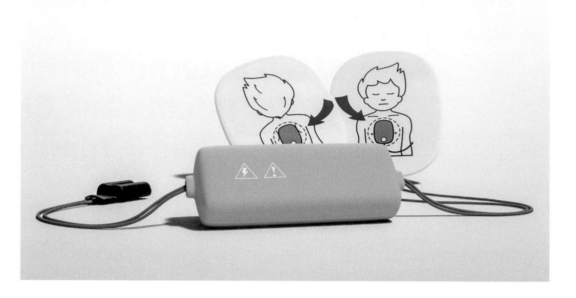

Choosing and Placing the AED Pads

Use child pads, if available, for infants and for children younger than 8 years of age. If child pads are not available, use adult pads. Make sure the pads do not touch each other or overlap. Adult pads deliver a higher shock dose, but a higher shock dose is better than no shock.

For pad placement, follow the AED manufacturer's instructions and the illustrations on the AED pads. Some AEDs require placing child pads in a front and back (anteroposterior [AP]) position (Figure 33), while others require right-left (anterolateral) placement. For infants, AP pad placement is common. See Critical Concepts: AED Pad Placement Options in Part 4.

Figure 33. AP AED pad placement on a child victim.

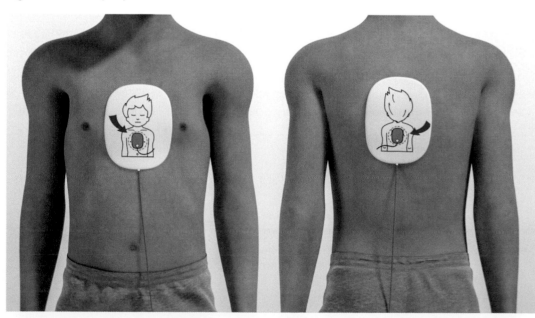

AED Use for Victims 8 Years of Age and Older

- Use the AED as soon as it is available.
- Use adult pads (Figure 34). **Do not use child pads**—they will likely give a shock dose that is too low.
- Place the pads as illustrated on the pads.
- Place the pads directly on the skin. Do not allow the pads to touch or overlap, and do not place on or over clothing.

AED Use for Victims Younger Than 8 Years of Age

- Use the AED as soon as it is available.
- Use child pads (Figure 35) if available. If you do not have child pads, you may use adult pads. Place the pads so that they do not touch each other.
- If the AED has a key or switch that will deliver a child shock dose, turn the key or switch.
- Place the pads as illustrated on the pads.
- Place the pads directly on the skin, and do not place on or over clothing.

Figure 34. Adult AED pads.

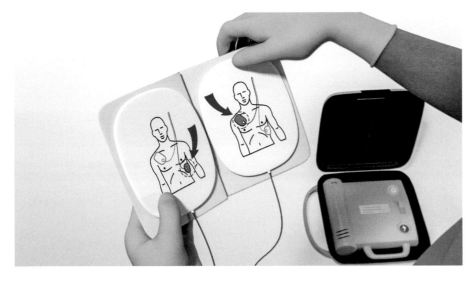

Figure 35. Child AED pads.

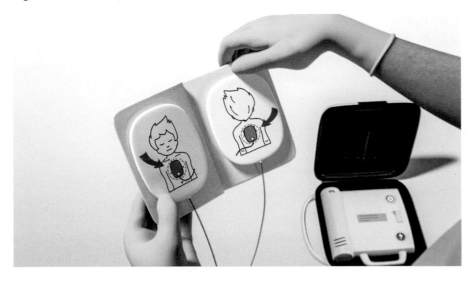

AED Use for Infants

For infants, a manual defibrillator is preferred to an AED. A manual defibrillator has more capabilities than an AED and can provide the lower energy doses that infants often need. This course does not cover how to use a manual defibrillator, a skill that requires advanced training.

- When a manual defibrillator is not available, an AED equipped with a pediatric dose attenuator is the preferred alternative.
- If neither is available, you may use an AED without a pediatric dose attenuator.

Critical Concepts:
Using Adult Pads or Adult Shock Dose Is Better Than No Defibrillation for an Infant or Child

AED Pads

If you are using an AED for an infant or for a child younger than 8 years of age and the AED does not have child pads, you may use adult pads. To ensure that the adult pads do not touch each other or overlap, you may need to place them anterior and posterior.

Shock Dose

If the AED you are using cannot deliver a pediatric dose, use the adult dose.

Review Questions

1. What should you do when using an AED on an infant or a child younger than 8 years of age?
   a. Never use adult AED pads.
   b. Use adult AED pads.
   c. Use adult AED pads if the AED does not have child pads.
   d. Use adult AED pads, but cut them in half.

2. If a manual defibrillator is not available for an infant victim, which action should you take?
   a. Perform high-quality CPR.
   b. Use an AED equipped with a pediatric dose attenuator.
   c. Cut the adult pad to fit the infant.
   d. Wait for advanced care to arrive.

3. What is important to remember about AED pad placement on infants?
   a. Ensure that pads overlap each other in very small infants.
   b. Place 1 adult pad on the chest.
   c. You may need to place 1 pad on the chest and 1 on the back, according to the diagrams on the pads.
   d. If child AED pads are not available, do not use the AED.

See Answers to Review Questions in the Appendix.

Part 8

Alternate Ventilation Techniques

As a BLS provider, you may be called on to help provide CPR in situations that require alternate ventilation techniques. If you are assisting advanced life support providers, you will need to know modifications to compressions and breaths once an advanced airway is placed. If a victim is unresponsive and not breathing but has a pulse, you will need to know how to perform rescue breathing. If a bag-mask device is not available, you may need to give mouth-to-mouth or mouth-to-nose breaths.

Learning Objectives

In this Part, you will learn about

- Modifications to compressions and breaths with an advanced airway in place
- Rescue breathing for respiratory arrest victims
- Techniques for giving breaths without a barrier device for adults, children, and infants

CPR and Breaths With an Advanced Airway

This section explains the modifications to compressions and breaths that rescuers must make when an advanced airway is in place. Advanced airways prevent airway obstruction and can provide a route for more effective oxygenation and ventilation. Examples of advanced airways are laryngeal mask airway, supraglottic airway device, and endotracheal tube.

Table 2 summarizes the compression-to-ventilation ratio with and without an advanced airway for adults, children, and infants.

Table 2. Compression-to-Ventilation Ratio During CPR With and Without an Advanced Airway

Ventilation technique	Compressions to breaths (adult)	Compressions to breaths (infant and child)
No advanced airway in place (eg, mouth-to-mouth, bag-mask device, pocket mask)	• Compression rate of 100-120/min • 30 compressions to 2 breaths	• Compression rate of 100-120/min • 30 compressions to 2 breaths (1 rescuer) • 15 compressions to 2 breaths (2 rescuers)

Advanced airway in place
 	
(eg, laryngeal mask airway, supraglottic airway device, endotracheal tube)
	• Compression rate of 100-120/min
	• Continuous compressions without pauses for breaths
	• Ventilation:
	  – Adult: 1 breath every 6 seconds
	  – Infant and child: 1 breath every 2-3 seconds	

Rescue Breathing

Rescue breathing is giving breaths to an unresponsive victim who has a pulse but is not breathing. You may provide rescue breathing by using a barrier device (eg, a pocket mask or face shield) or a bag-mask device. If emergency equipment is not available, you may provide breaths by using the mouth-to-mouth technique or the mouth-to-mouth-and-nose technique.

How to Provide Rescue Breathing for Adults, Infants, and Children

- **For adults:**
  - Give **1 breath every 6 seconds**.
  - Give each breath over 1 second.
  - Each breath should result in visible chest rise.
  - Check for a pulse about every 2 minutes.
- **For infants and children**:
  - Give **1 breath every 2 to 3 seconds**.
  - Give each breath over 1 second.
  - Each breath should result in visible chest rise.
  - Check for a pulse about every 2 minutes.

When to Switch From Only Rescue Breathing to CPR in an Infant or a Child

When you are providing rescue breathing only, start CPR (compressions *and* breaths) if you see the following:

- Signs of poor perfusion in an infant despite effective oxygenation and ventilation provided by rescue breathing
- The infant's or child's heart rate is less than 60/min with signs of poor perfusion
- When a pulse is no longer felt

Critical Concepts:
Respiratory Arrest

- Respiratory arrest occurs when normal breathing stops, preventing essential oxygen supply and carbon dioxide exchange. Lack of oxygen to the brain eventually causes a person to become unresponsive.
- Rescuers can identify respiratory arrest if all of the following signs are present:
    - The victim is unresponsive
    - The victim is not breathing or is only gasping
    - The victim still has a pulse
- Respiratory arrest is an emergency. Without immediate treatment, it can result in brain injury, cardiac arrest, and death.
- In certain situations, including opioid-associated life-threatening emergencies, respiratory arrest is potentially reversible if rescuers treat it early. (See Part 9 for more about opioids.)
- BLS providers must be able to quickly identify respiratory arrest, activate the emergency response system, and begin rescue breathing. Quick action can prevent the development of cardiac arrest.

Techniques for Giving Breaths Without a Barrier Device

Many cardiac arrests happen in settings where rescue equipment is not available. This section describes techniques for giving breaths when you do not have a barrier device, such as a pocket mask or a bag-mask device.

Mouth-to-Mouth Breathing for Adults and Children

Mouth-to-mouth breathing is a quick, effective technique to provide oxygen to an unresponsive adult or child. Follow these steps to give mouth-to-mouth breaths to adults and children:

1. Hold the victim's airway open with a head tilt–chin lift.
2. Pinch the nose closed with your thumb and index finger (using the hand on the forehead).
3. Take a regular (not deep) breath and seal your lips around the victim's mouth, creating an airtight seal (Figure 36).
4. Deliver 1 breath over 1 second. Watch for the chest to rise as you give the breath.
5. If the chest does not rise, repeat the head tilt–chin lift.
6. Give a second breath (blow for about 1 second). Watch for the chest to rise.
7. If you are unable to ventilate the victim after 2 attempts, promptly return to chest compressions.

Figure 36. Mouth-to-mouth breaths.

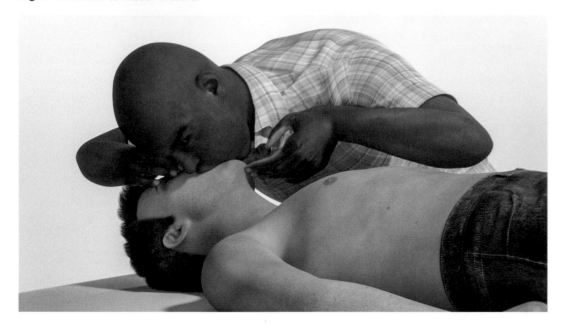

Breathing Techniques for Infants

Use one of the following techniques to give breaths in infants:

- Mouth-to-mouth-and-nose
- Mouth-to-mouth

The preferred technique for infants is mouth-to-mouth-and-nose. However, if you cannot cover the infant's nose and mouth with your mouth, use the mouth-to-mouth technique instead.

Mouth-to-Mouth-and-Nose Technique

1. Maintain a head tilt–chin lift to keep the airway open.
2. Place your mouth over the infant's mouth and nose and create an airtight seal (Figure 37).
3. Blow into the infant's nose and mouth (pausing to inhale between breaths), just enough to make the chest rise with each breath.
4. If the chest does not rise, repeat the head tilt–chin lift to reopen the airway, and then try again to give a breath that makes the chest rise. It may be necessary to move the infant's head through a range of positions to provide effective breaths. When the airway is open, give breaths that make the chest rise.

Mouth-to-Mouth Technique

1. Maintain a head tilt–chin lift to keep the airway open.
2. Pinch the victim's nose tightly with your thumb and forefinger.
3. Make a mouth-to-mouth seal.
4. Deliver each mouth-to-mouth breath, making sure the chest rises with each breath.
5. If the chest does not rise, repeat the head tilt–chin lift to reopen the airway. It may be necessary to move the infant's head through a range of positions to provide effective breaths. When the airway is open, give breaths that make the chest rise.

Figure 37. Mouth-to-mouth-and-nose breaths for an infant victim.

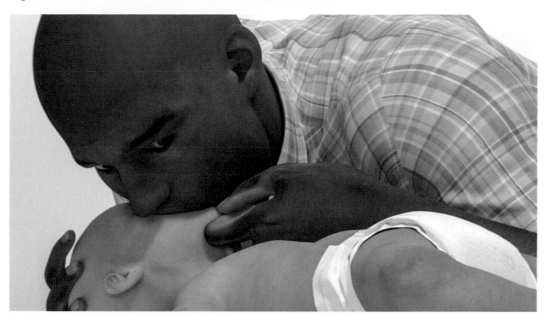

Caution: Risk of Gastric Inflation

If you give breaths too quickly or with too much force, air is likely to enter the stomach rather than the lungs. This can cause *gastric inflation* (filling of the stomach with air).

Gastric inflation frequently develops during mouth-to-mouth, mouth-to-mask, or bag-mask ventilation. It can result in serious complications. To reduce the risk of gastric inflation, avoid giving breaths too quickly, too forcefully, or with too much volume. But even if you give breaths correctly during high-quality CPR, gastric inflation may still develop.

To reduce the risk of gastric inflation

- Deliver each breath over 1 second
- Deliver just enough air to make the victim's chest rise

Review Questions

1. Which victim would need only rescue breathing?
   a. Agonal gasping with no pulse
   b. Breathing with a weak pulse
   c. No breathing and a pulse
   d. No breathing and no pulse

2. How often should rescue breaths be given in infants and children when a pulse is felt?
   a. 1 breath every 2 to 3 seconds
   b. 1 breath every 3 to 5 seconds
   c. 1 breath every 5 to 6 seconds
   d. 1 breath every 8 to 10 seconds

3. Which action can rescuers perform to potentially reduce the risk of gastric inflation?
   a. Delivering each breath over 1 second
   b. Giving rapid, shallow breaths
   c. Using a bag-mask device for delivering ventilation
   d. Using the mouth-to-mask breathing technique

4. Which is the preferred technique for giving rescue breaths to an infant?

   a. Mouth-to-mouth
   b. Mouth-to-mouth-and-nose
   c. Mouth-to-nose
   d. Any method is acceptable

See Answers to Review Questions in the Appendix.

Part 9

Opioid-Associated Life-Threatening Emergencies

Deaths related to opioid use are increasing. The World Health Organization estimates that 27 million people suffer from opioid use disorders. Most use illicit drugs, but an increasing number are using prescribed opioids. In the United States, drug overdose involving opioids is a leading cause of injury-related death. About 130 Americans die every day from an opioid overdose. Opioid overdose does not just occur in addicts; it can occur in anyone who takes opioids or has access to opioids. Unintentional overdose can happen at any time, to any person, of any age, and in any place.

Given this ongoing crisis, it is important to know what to do if you suspect an opioid-associated life-threatening emergency (opioid drug overdose) in an unresponsive adult victim.

Learning Objectives

In this Part, you will learn

- How to recognize an opioid-associated life-threatening emergency
- The importance of administering naloxone in opioid-associated life-threatening emergencies
- The steps in the opioid-associated life-threatening emergency response sequence

What Are Opioids?

Opioids are medications used primarily for pain relief. Common examples are hydrocodone, morphine, and fentanyl. Heroin is an example of an opioid that is illegal in the United States.

Problematic Opioid Use

Many people think that problematic opioid use happens only when someone takes an illegally produced or obtained opioid. Yet problems can occur when someone

- Takes more drug than is prescribed (either purposely or accidentally)
- Takes an opioid that was prescribed for someone else
- Combines opioids with alcohol or certain other drugs, such as tranquilizers or sleeping pills
- Has certain medical conditions, such as reduced liver function or sleep apnea
- Is older than 65 years of age

Too much opioid in the body can overwhelm the brain and depress the natural drive to breathe. This respiratory depression can result in respiratory arrest and cardiac arrest.

Identifying an Opioid Emergency

Scene Assessment

Scene assessment is an important tool for identifying whether opioids may be involved in a life-threatening emergency. To evaluate the scene for potential opioid overdose, use these strategies:

- Communicate with bystanders: Ask questions such as, "Does anyone have any information about what happened? Do you know if the victim took anything?"
- Observe the victim: Look for signs of injection on the skin, a medication patch, or other signs of opioid use.
- Assess the surroundings: Look for medication bottles or other signs of opioid use.

Signs of an Opioid Overdose

Look for the following signs of an opioid overdose:

- Slow, shallow, or no breathing
- Choking or gurgling sounds
- Drowsiness or loss of consciousness
- Small, constricted pupils
- Blue skin, lips, or nails

Do not delay lifesaving actions. After confirming scene safety, rescuers may perform the assessment at the same time as the resuscitation attempt.

Antidote to Opioid Overdose: Naloxone

The drug naloxone can temporarily reverse the effects of respiratory depression that opioids can cause. If available, give naloxone quickly by one of these delivery routes: intramuscular, intranasal, or intravenous (given by advanced providers).

Naloxone Autoinjector

Naloxone handheld autoinjectors deliver a single dose via an intramuscular injection.

Intranasal Naloxone

An easy-to-use atomizer device delivers intranasal naloxone into the nose. There is no risk of needle-stick injuries with this method. The body quickly absorbs intranasal naloxone because the nasal cavity has a relatively large surface of mucus membranes rich in capillaries.

Critical Concepts:
What to Do for an Opioid-Associated Life-Threatening Emergency

If you suspect an opioid-associated life-threatening emergency, do the following:

- ***If the victim has a definite pulse but is not breathing normally****: Provide rescue breaths and give naloxone according to package directions and per local protocol. Monitor for response.*
- ***If the victim is in cardiac arrest and you suspect an opioid overdose****: Start CPR. Consider giving naloxone per package directions and per local protocol. Note that for victims who are in cardiac arrest from opioid overdose, the effect of administering naloxone is not known.*

Opioid-Associated Life-Threatening Emergency Response Sequence

The first rescuer who arrives at the side of an unresponsive victim and suspects opioid use should quickly follow these steps. *As with any life-threatening emergency, do not delay lifesaving actions.*

Step 1: If you suspect opioid poisoning:

- Check to see if the person responds.
- Shout for nearby help.
- Activate the emergency response system.
- If you are alone, get naloxone and an AED if available. If someone else is present, send that person to get them.

Step 2: Is the person breathing normally?

- If the person is breathing normally, proceed with Steps 3 and 4.
- If the person is not breathing normally, go to Step 5.

Step 3: Prevent deterioration.

- Tap and shout. Check for responsiveness by tapping the victim's shoulders. Shout, "Are you OK?"
- Open and reposition the airway if needed to maintain normal breathing. This may be necessary if the victim is unresponsive or is responsive but unable to maintain an open airway due to a depressed level of consciousness.
- Consider administering naloxone, if available. If you suspect an opioid overdose, it is reasonable to give naloxone according to package directions and per local protocol. Monitor for response.
- Transport to the hospital. If the victim is not already in a healthcare setting, they should be transported by EMS to a hospital.

Step 4: Assess for responsiveness and breathing.

Continue to assess responsiveness and breathing until the victim is transferred to advanced care. Victims with opioid-associated emergencies may not be able to maintain an open airway or breathe normally. Even those who receive naloxone may develop respiratory problems that can lead to cardiac arrest.

Step 5: Does the person have a pulse?

Assess for a pulse for no more than 10 seconds.

- If yes (a pulse is felt), go to Step 6.
- If no (a pulse is not felt), go to Step 7.

Step 6: Support ventilation.

- Open and reposition the airway before giving rescue breaths.
- Provide rescue breathing or bag-mask ventilation. This can help prevent cardiac arrest. Continue until spontaneous, normal breathing occurs. Reassess the victim's breathing and pulse every 2 minutes. If there is no pulse, provide CPR (see Step 7).
- Give naloxone according to package directions and per local protocol.

Step 7: Start CPR.

- If the victim is not breathing normally and no pulse is felt, provide high-quality CPR, including ventilation. Use the AED as soon as it is available.
- Consider naloxone. If naloxone is available and you suspect an opioid overdose, it is reasonable to give it according to package directions and per local protocol. High-quality CPR should take priority over giving naloxone.
- Refer to the BLS protocol (see Figure 4).

For more information, see Figure 45 in the Appendix.

Review Questions

1. Which of these is not an opioid?
   a. Heroin
   b. Hydrocodone
   c. Morphine
   d. Naloxone

2. Your roommate uses opioids. You find him unresponsive with no breathing, but he has a strong pulse. You suspect an opioid overdose. A friend is phoning 9-1-1 and looking for the naloxone autoinjector. What action should you take?
   a. Remain with your roommate until the naloxone arrives and administer it immediately.
   b. Begin CPR, starting with chest compressions.
   c. Provide rescue breathing: 1 breath every 6 seconds.
   d. Provide rapid defibrillation with an AED.

3. You encounter an unresponsive 56-year-old woman who has been taking hydrocodone for postsurgical pain. She is not breathing and has no pulse. You notice that her medication bottle is empty and suspect an opioid-associated life-threatening emergency. A colleague activates the emergency response system and is retrieving the AED and naloxone. What is the most appropriate action for you to take next?
   a. Wait for the naloxone to arrive before doing anything.
   b. Begin CPR, starting with chest compressions.
   c. Provide 1 rescue breath every 6 seconds until naloxone arrives.
   d. Provide rapid defibrillation with the AED.

See Answers to Review Questions in the Appendix.

Other Life-Threatening Emergencies

BLS providers may be called to respond to life-threatening medical emergencies that have not yet progressed to cardiac arrest. Some of these emergencies are heart attack, stroke, drowning, and anaphylaxis. You may save a life by recognizing what needs to be done and acting quickly.

Learning Objectives

At the end of this Part, you will be able to

- Recognize signs of heart attack and describe actions to help a heart attack victim
- Recognize signs of stroke and describe actions to help a stroke victim
- Discuss examples of how to tailor rescue actions based on the cause of cardiac arrest
- Describe actions to help a victim of cardiac arrest due to drowning
- Describe signs of a severe allergic reaction and the criteria for anaphylaxis
- Describe actions to help someone with a severe allergic reaction
- Discuss how to use an epinephrine autoinjector

Heart Attack

Heart disease has been the leading cause of death in the United States for both men and women for decades. Every 40 seconds, a person in the United States has a heart attack.

A heart attack occurs when a blockage forms or there is a severe spasm in a blood vessel that restricts the flow of blood and oxygen to the heart muscle. During a heart attack, the heart typically continues to pump blood. But the longer the victim with a heart attack goes without treatment to restore blood flow, the greater the possible damage to the heart muscle. Sometimes, the damaged heart muscle triggers an abnormal rhythm that can lead to sudden cardiac arrest.

Signs of Heart Attack

Signs of a heart attack may occur suddenly and be intense. Yet many heart attacks start slowly with mild pain or discomfort. Activate the emergency response system if someone is having signs of heart attack (Figure 38):

- **Chest discomfort.** Most heart attacks involve discomfort in the center of the chest that lasts more than a few minutes and often does not resolve with rest. The discomfort may go away with rest and then return. It can feel like uncomfortable pressure, squeezing, fullness, or pain.

- **Discomfort in other areas of the upper body.** Symptoms can include pain or discomfort in the left arm (commonly) but can occur in both arms, the upper back, neck, jaw, or stomach.
- **Shortness of breath.** This can occur with or without chest discomfort.
- **Other signs.** Breaking out in a cold sweat, nausea, vomiting, or light-headedness are other signs.

The typical signs of a heart attack are based on the experience of white, middle-aged men. Women, the elderly, and people with diabetes are more likely to have less typical signs of a heart attack, such as shortness of breath, weakness, unusual fatigue, cold sweat, and dizziness. Women who report chest discomfort may describe it as pressure, aching, or tightness rather than as pain.

Other less typical signs are heartburn or indigestion; an uncomfortable feeling in the back, jaw, neck, or shoulder; and nausea or vomiting. People who have trouble communicating may not be able to articulate signs of a heart attack.

Figure 38. Common heart attack warning signs.

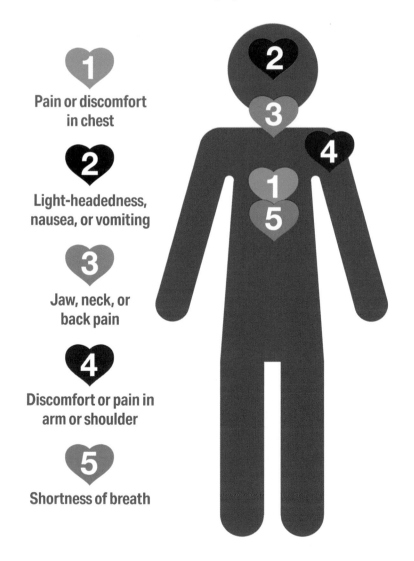

1. Pain or discomfort in chest

2. Light-headedness, nausea, or vomiting

3. Jaw, neck, or back pain

4. Discomfort or pain in arm or shoulder

5. Shortness of breath

Heart Attack and Sudden Cardiac Arrest

People often use the terms *heart attack* and *cardiac arrest* to mean the same thing, but they are not the same.

- A *heart attack* is a blood flow problem. It occurs because a blockage or spasm in a blood vessel severely restricts or cuts off the flow of blood and oxygen to the heart muscle.
- *Sudden cardiac arrest* is usually a rhythm problem. It occurs when the heart develops an abnormal rhythm. This abnormal rhythm causes the heart to quiver—or stop completely— and no longer pump blood to the brain, lungs, and other organs.

Within seconds, a victim in cardiac arrest becomes unresponsive and is not breathing or is only gasping. Death occurs within minutes if the victim does not receive immediate lifesaving treatment.

Heart attack happens more frequently than cardiac arrest. Although most heart attacks do not lead to cardiac arrest, they are a common cause. Other conditions that change the heart's rhythm may lead to cardiac arrest also.

Obstacles to Lifesaving Treatment

Early recognition, early intervention, and early transport of someone with a suspected heart attack is critical. Early access to the EMS system is often delayed because both the victim and bystanders fail to recognize the signs of a heart attack. Lifesaving treatment can be delivered by emergency medical providers on the way to the hospital, saving precious minutes and heart muscle.

Many people won't admit that their discomfort may be caused by a heart attack. People often say the following:

- "I'm too healthy" or "I'm too young."
- "I don't want to bother the doctor."
- "I don't want to frighten my spouse."
- "I'll feel silly if it isn't a heart attack."
- "It's just indigestion."

If you suspect someone is having a heart attack, act quickly and activate the emergency response system. Don't hesitate, even if the victim doesn't want to admit discomfort.

Actions to Help a Heart Attack Victim

Heart attack is a time-critical emergency. Every minute counts. If you think someone is having a heart attack, do the following:

1. Have the victim sit and remain calm.
2. Activate the emergency response system or ask someone else to do so. Get the first aid kit and AED if available.
3. Encourage alert adults who are experiencing chest pain to chew and swallow aspirin unless they have a known aspirin allergy or have been told not to take aspirin by a healthcare provider.
4. If the victim becomes unresponsive and is not breathing or is only gasping, start CPR.

System of Care

Effective treatment of heart attack requires a well-coordinated, timely system of care. "Time is muscle!" Every minute counts. The longer a heart attack victim waits for treatment, the more damage to the heart muscle. Timely interventions by healthcare providers in the hospital to open the blocked coronary blood vessel can determine the amount of damage to the heart muscle. One common intervention is nonsurgical treatment in the cardiac cath lab. Administration of an intravenous medication in the ED is another intervention.

Actions of healthcare providers during the first several hours of a heart attack determine how much the patient will benefit from treatment. The goal is to decrease time from symptom onset until the blockage is resolved.

Here are the steps in the out-of-hospital system of care for heart attack:

- **Early recognition and call for help.** The more quickly first responders or family recognize the warning signs of heart attack, the sooner treatment can begin. The emergency response system should be activated immediately for triage and transport. Family members should not drive the suspected heart attack victim to the hospital. Victims should not drive themselves. Emergency responders can provide some interventions at the scene or during transport, thus lessening delay to definitive treatment in the hospital.
- **Early EMS evaluation and 12-lead ECG.** The 12-lead ECG is the central component for triage of patients with chest discomfort. When EMS providers are able to perform a 12-lead ECG and transmit results to the receiving hospital, time to treatment is decreased. The ECG may be done at the scene or during transport.
- **Early heart attack identification.** Once providers confirm a heart attack, they communicate with advanced care providers and transport the patient to the most appropriate hospital.
- **Early notification.** EMS providers notify the receiving facility as soon as possible of an incoming heart attack patient. The cath lab team is activated before the patient's arrival. EMS activation of the cardiac cath lab speeds the time to diagnosis and intervention.
- **Early intervention.** The goal time from initial contact to treatment interventions is less than 90 minutes.

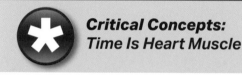

Critical Concepts:
Time Is Heart Muscle

- *Early recognition, early EMS activation, early transport by EMS, and early intervention for someone with a suspected heart attack is critical. The goal is 90 minutes from initial contact to treatment intervention.*
- *Learn to recognize the signs of a heart attack. Activate the emergency response system without delay. Give aspirin if indicated. Be prepared to start CPR if the victim becomes unresponsive.*

Stroke

Every 40 seconds, someone in the United States has a stroke. More than 795 000 people have a stroke every year. Stroke is a leading cause of serious long-term disability and the fifth leading cause of death.

A stroke occurs when blood stops flowing to a part of the brain. This can happen if an artery in the brain is blocked (ischemic stroke) or a blood vessel bursts (hemorrhagic stroke). Brain cells begin to die within minutes without blood and oxygen. Treatment in the first hours after a stroke can reduce damage to the brain and improve recovery.

Warning Signs of Stroke

Use the F.A.S.T. method to recognize and remember the warning signs of stroke (Table 3). F.A.S.T. stands for face drooping, arm weakness, speech difficulty, and time to phone 9-1-1. If you see any of these signs, act F.A.S.T.

Table 3. Spot a Stroke F.A.S.T.

Letter	Stroke warning signs
F	**Face drooping:** Does one side of the face droop or is it numb? Ask the person to smile.
A	**Arm weakness:** Is one arm weak or numb? Ask the person to raise both arms. Does one arm drift downward?
S	**Speech difficulty:** Is speech slurred? Is the victim unable to speak or hard to understand? Ask the person to repeat a simple sentence, like "The sky is blue." Is the sentence repeated correctly?
T	**Time to phone 9-1-1:** If the person shows any of these symptoms, even if the symptoms go away, phone 9-1-1 and get them to the hospital immediately.

Other Signs of Stroke

Be alert for other common signs of stroke, such as

- Sudden dizziness, trouble walking, or loss of balance or coordination
- Sudden trouble seeing in one or both eyes
- Sudden severe headache with no known cause
- Sudden numbness of the face, arm, or leg
- Sudden weakness in part of the body
- Sudden confusion or trouble understanding others

Actions to Help a Stroke Victim

Stroke is a time-critical emergency. Every minute counts. If you think someone has had a stroke, do the following:

1. Quickly evaluate the victim for signs of stroke.
2. Activate the emergency response system or have someone else do so.
3. Find out what time the signs of stroke first appeared.
4. Remain with the victim until someone with more advanced training arrives and takes over.
5. If the victim becomes unresponsive and is not breathing normally or is only gasping, give CPR.

System of Care

Effective stroke treatment requires a well-coordinated, timely system of care. Delay at any step limits treatment options. The longer a stroke patient waits for treatment, the more brain tissue dies. Drugs that break up a clot must be given within about 3 hours after the time the signs first started. Providers must know the last-known-well time. This is the point at which the patient was last known to be well without signs of stroke.

Here are the steps in the out-of-hospital system of care for stroke:

1. **Recognition.** The more quickly first responders or family recognize the warning signs of stroke (Table 3), the sooner treatment can begin. Patients who do not get to the ED within a 3-hour window, from the onset of symptoms, may not be eligible for certain types of therapy.
2. **EMS dispatch.** Someone should phone 9-1-1 and get EMS on the way as quickly as possible. Family members should not transport the stroke victim to the hospital themselves.
3. **EMS identification, management, and transport.** EMS will determine if the patient is showing signs of a stroke and obtain important medical history. They will begin management and transport to the next level of care. EMS will call ahead to the receiving hospital to alert providers that a potential stroke patient will soon be arriving.
4. **Triage.** The patient should be triaged to the closest available stroke center or hospital that provides emergency stroke care.

5. **Evaluation and management.** Once the patient arrives at the ED, evaluation and management should proceed immediately.

6. **Treatment decisions.** Providers with stroke expertise will determine appropriate therapy.

7. **Therapy.** The gold standard treatment for ischemic stroke is an intravenous administration of alteplase. To be effective, alteplase must be given within about 3 hours after the time the signs first started. Another option is thrombectomy, an invasive procedure that removes the clot from inside the blood vessel or artery.

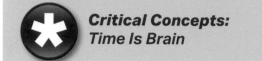

Critical Concepts:
Time Is Brain

Stroke is a time-critical emergency. Every minute treatment is delayed, more brain tissue dies. Priorities are early recognition, limited scene time, and transport to the appropriate facility.

Drowning

Drowning is the third leading cause of injury death worldwide. In the United States, drowning is the second leading cause of injury death for children ages 1 to 14. Nonfatal drowning injuries can cause severe brain damage, resulting in disabilities and permanent loss of basic functioning.

Rescue Actions Based on Cause of Cardiac Arrest

BLS providers may need to tailor rescue actions to the most likely cause of arrest. For example, if you are alone and see someone suddenly collapse, then it is reasonable to assume that the victim has had a sudden cardiac arrest. The steps for a sudden cardiac arrest are to activate the emergency response system, get an AED, and then return to the victim to provide CPR. CPR for a victim of sudden cardiac arrest begins with chest compressions. The sequence for a victim of drowning is different. Cardiac arrest in a drowning victim is caused by a severe lack of oxygen in the body (asphyxial arrest). The priority is to get oxygen to the brain, heart, and other tissues.

Actions to Help a Victim of Cardiac Arrest Due to Drowning

Follow these steps along with the Adult BLS for Healthcare Providers algorithm to help a victim of cardiac arrest:

1. **Call for help.** Ask someone to activate the emergency response system. Get to the victim as quickly as possible. Move the victim to shallow water or out of the water. Pay attention to your own personal safety during the rescue process.

2. **Check for breathing.** If there is no breathing, open the airway. Give 2 rescue breaths that make the chest rise. Avoid delays in beginning CPR. Use mouth-to-nose ventilation as an alternative to mouth-to-mouth ventilation if needed. Sometimes it is difficult for the rescuer to pinch the victim's nose, support the head, and open the airway if the victim is still in the water.

   a. You do not need to perform routine spinal stabilization unless there are signs that the victim may have a head or neck injury.

   b. Do not try to clear the airway of aspirated water. Most drowning victims only aspirate a modest amount of water, and it is absorbed rapidly.

   c. Do not use abdominal thrusts to try to remove water from the breathing passages. These actions are not recommended and can be dangerous.

3. Check for a pulse after giving 2 effective breaths.

   a. If the victim is not breathing normally but has a pulse, provide rescue breathing only. Recheck for a pulse every 2 minutes.

   b. If you do not feel a pulse, start CPR.

4. Start CPR with cycles of 30 compressions and 2 breaths. Give 5 cycles (about 2 minutes) and then activate the emergency response system if not already done.

5. Use the AED as soon as it is available. Attach the AED once the victim is out of the water. You only need to dry the chest area quickly before applying the AED pads.

6. Follow the AED prompts. If no shock is needed and after any shock delivery, immediately resume CPR, starting with chest compressions.

Vomiting During Resuscitation

The victim may vomit during rescue breaths or chest compressions. If this happens, turn the victim to the side. If you suspect a spinal cord injury, roll the victim so that the head, neck, and torso are turned as a unit. This will help protect the cervical spine. Remove the vomit using your finger or a cloth. You may use suction if within your scope of practice.

Transport

All victims of drowning should be transported by EMS to the ED for evaluation and monitoring. This includes victims who needed only rescue breaths or those who are alert and seem to have recovered. Although survival is uncommon in victims who have been underwater for a long time, there have been cases of successful recovery, especially when in cold water. For this reason, rescuers should provide CPR at the scene, and the victim should be transported in accordance with local protocols.

Critical Concepts:
Rescue Breaths First

The first and most important action for a drowning victim is to give rescue breaths as soon as possible. This action increases the victim's chance of survival.

Anaphylaxis

Most allergic reactions are mild. Some, however, worsen to a state of anaphylaxis. Anaphylaxis is a severe allergic reaction that requires urgent treatment. Treatment may include an epinephrine injection.

Prompt recognition is critical. You must be able to identify if an allergic reaction is mild or severe (anaphylaxis).

Mild Allergic Reaction

Signs of a Mild Allergic Reaction

Signs of a mild allergic reaction are

- Stuffy nose, sneezing, and itching around the eyes
- Itching of the skin or mucous membranes
- Raised, red rash on the skin (hives)

Actions for Mild Allergic Reaction

- Get help.
- Remove the victim from the allergen if known (move out of the environment, wash the affected area of skin).
- Ask about any history of allergy or anaphylaxis; look for a medical alert bracelet or necklace.
- Consider an oral dose of antihistamine.

Severe Allergic Reaction

A severe allergic reaction (anaphylaxis) can be life threatening if not recognized and treated immediately. Anaphylaxis occurs suddenly after contact with an allergen. Some common allergens associated with anaphylaxis are medicines, latex, foods, and stinging insects. In anaphylaxis, 2 or more body systems are involved.

Signs of a Severe Allergic Reaction

Signs of a severe allergic reaction may include

- **Breathing.** Swelling of the airway, trouble breathing, and abnormal breathing sounds (such as wheezing)
- **Skin.** Hives, itching, flushing, and swelling of the lips, tongue, and face
- **Circulation.** Signs of poor perfusion (shock), which may include very fast heart rate, changes in skin color, cool skin, not alert, low blood pressure
- **Gastrointestinal.** Stomach cramping, diarrhea

Criteria for Anaphylaxis

Many providers have trouble recognizing anaphylaxis. Look for the following 4 criteria:

- Signs that come on quickly and rapidly get worse
- Skin changes, such as flushing, itching, and swelling of the lips, tongue, and face
- Life-threatening airway, breathing, or circulation problems
- Involvement of 2 or more body systems

Remember that skin changes alone are not a sign of an anaphylactic reaction.

Epinephrine Autoinjector for a Severe Allergic Reaction

Epinephrine is a drug that can temporarily relieve the life-threatening problems caused by a severe allergic reaction. It is available by prescription in a self-injectable device called an epinephrine autoinjector. People who are known to have severe allergic reactions are encouraged to carry epinephrine autoinjectors with them at all times.

There are 2 types of epinephrine autoinjectors: spring activated and electronic. Doses are different for children and adults. The epinephrine injection is given in the side of the thigh, about halfway between the hip and the knee (Figure 39B). This is the safest location for administration. Epinephrine can be given on bare skin or through clothing.

Someone who has an epinephrine autoinjector will generally know how and when to use it. If the person is unable, you may help give the injection if the medication has been prescribed by a physician and state law permits it.

Actions to Help Someone With a Severe Allergic Reaction

A severe allergic reaction can be life threatening. Follow these steps to help someone with suspected anaphylaxis:

1. Activate the emergency response system or ask someone else to do so. Send someone to get the person's epinephrine autoinjector(s).
2. Give or help the person inject epinephrine with an epinephrine autoinjector as soon as possible (Figure 39). See How to Use an Epinephrine Autoinjector.
3. Send someone to get the AED.

4. Give a second dose of epinephrine if the person has continued symptoms and advanced care will not arrive in 5 to 10 minutes.

5. If the person becomes unresponsive and is not breathing or is only gasping, start CPR. You may give epinephrine by epinephrine autoinjector during cardiac arrest.

6. If possible, save a sample of what caused the reaction. Give it to the advanced responders.

Critical Concepts:
Lifesaving Action for Anaphylaxis

The first and most important action for someone with suspected anaphylaxis is to give an immediate injection of epinephrine using their epinephrine autoinjector.

How to Use an Epinephrine Autoinjector

You should know the correct technique for using an epinephrine autoinjector. Some devices give voice prompts to guide users through the administration of the epinephrine dose.

Device Safety

Before using the epinephrine autoinjector, quickly examine it to make sure it is safe to use. Do not use it if the

- Solution is discolored (when it is possible to see the medicine)
- Clear window on the autoinjector is red

Steps for Using an Epinephrine Autoinjector

Follow these steps to correctly use an epinephrine autoinjector:

1. Follow the instructions on the device. Make sure you are holding the device in your fist without touching either end because the needle comes out of one end. You may give the injection through clothes or on bare skin. Take off the safety cap (Figure 39A).

2. Hold the leg firmly in place just before and during the injection. Press the tip of the injector hard against the side of the person's thigh, about halfway between the hip and the knee (Figure 39B).

3. For EpiPen and EpiPen Jr injectors, hold the injector in place for 3 seconds. Some other injectors may be held in place for up to 10 seconds. Be familiar with the manufacturer's instructions for the type of injector you are using.

4. Pull the injector straight out, making sure you do not put your fingers over the end that has been pressed against the person's thigh.

5. Either the person getting the injection or the one giving the injection should rub the injection spot for about 10 seconds.

6. Note the time of the injection. Properly dispose of the injector.

7. Ensure that EMS is on the way. If there is a delay greater than 5 to 10 minutes for advanced help to arrive, consider giving a second dose, if available.

Figure 39. Using an epinephrine autoinjector. **A,** Take off the safety cap. **B,** Press the tip of the injector hard against the side of the thigh, about halfway between the hip and the knee.

A

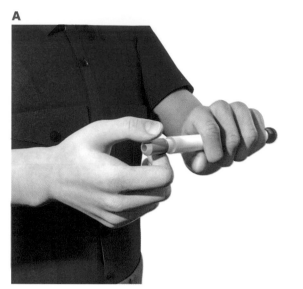

B

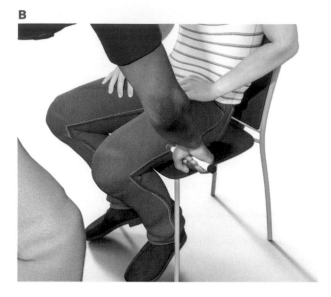

Safe Disposal

It's important to dispose of used needles correctly so that no one gets stuck. Follow the sharps disposal policy at your workplace. If you don't know what to do with the used injector, give it to someone with more advanced training.

Review Questions

1. Which of the following populations is most likely to show atypical signs of a heart attack, like shortness of breath and dizziness?
   a. White, middle-aged men
   b. Individuals with diabetes
   c. Younger-aged individuals
   d. People who are overweight

2. What does the stroke acronym F.A.S.T. stand for?
   a. Face drooping, arm weakness, speech difficulty, time to phone 9-1-1
   b. Falling down, arm weakness, slurring words, time to start first aid
   c. Falling down, arm tingling, speech difficulty, time to phone 9-1-1
   d. Face drooping, arm tingling, sudden weakness, time to start CPR

3. If you think someone might be having a stroke, what should be the first thing you do?
   a. Start first aid on the individual.
   b. Wait an hour and then phone 9-1-1.
   c. Give the person an injection of alteplase.
   d. Quickly check for signs of stroke.

4. How are rescue actions for cardiac arrest due to drowning different from the rescue actions for sudden cardiac arrest?
   a. Unlike sudden cardiac arrest, the priority in a drowning is to give the person CPR.
   b. Unlike sudden cardiac arrest, the priority in a drowning is to give the person oxygen.
   c. Unlike sudden cardiac arrest, the priority in a drowning is to locate an ambulance.
   d. Unlike sudden cardiac arrest, the priority in a drowning is to give chest compressions.

5. You are attempting to rescue a person who has experienced drowning. What do you do if there are no signs of breathing?

    a. Attempt to clear the airway of aspirated water.

    b. Perform abdominal thrusts to remove any water.

    c. Open the airway and administer rescue breaths.

    d. Use spinal stabilization regardless of neck injury.

6. Which of the following is a sign that someone is experiencing anaphylaxis?

    a. Symptoms developing quickly but getting worse slowly

    b. Presence of a medical alert bracelet or necklace

    c. Person responding well to oral antihistamines

    d. Life-threatening breathing or circulation problems

7. You notice someone showing all the signs of a severe allergic reaction. What is the first and most important action you should take?

    a. Call an advanced responder.

    b. Use the epinephrine device.

    c. Give the person an oral antihistamine.

    d. Locate an external defibrillator.

8. Where on the body should you administer an epinephrine injection?

    a. On the person's thigh, about halfway between the hip and the knee

    b. On the person's torso, about halfway between the hip and the ribs

    c. On the person's arm, about halfway between the elbow and the wrist

    d. On the person's neck, about halfway between the ear and the shoulder

See Answers to Review Questions in the Appendix.

Part 11

Choking Relief for Adults, Children, and Infants

This section discusses how to recognize choking (foreign-body airway obstruction) and then perform maneuvers to relieve the obstruction. Choking relief maneuvers are the same for adults and children (1 year of age and older). You will learn a different technique to relieve choking for infants (younger than 1 year of age).

Learning Objectives

In this Part, you will learn

- The technique for relief of foreign-body airway obstruction for an adult or child
- The technique for relief of foreign-body airway obstruction for an infant

Signs of Choking

Early recognition of foreign-body airway obstruction is the key to successful outcome. It is important to distinguish this emergency from fainting, stroke, heart attack, seizure, drug overdose, or other conditions that may cause sudden respiratory distress but require different treatment.

Foreign bodies may cause a range of signs from *mild* to *severe* airway obstruction (Table 4).

Table 4. Signs of Foreign-Body Airway Obstruction and Rescuer Actions

Type of obstruction	Signs	Rescuer actions
Mild airway obstruction	• Good air exchange • Can cough forcefully • May wheeze between coughs	• As long as good air exchange continues, encourage the victim to continue coughing. • Do not interfere with the victim's own attempts to relieve the obstruction. Stay with the victim and monitor the condition. • If mild airway obstruction continues or progresses to signs of severe airway obstruction, activate the emergency response system.
Severe airway obstruction	• Clutching the throat with the thumb and fingers, making the universal choking sign (Figure 40) • Unable to speak or cry • Poor or no air exchange • Weak, ineffective cough or no cough at all • High-pitched noise while inhaling or no noise at all • Increased respiratory difficulty • Possible cyanosis (blue lips or skin)	• If the victim is an adult or child, ask "Are you choking?" If the victim nods "yes" and cannot talk, severe airway obstruction is present. • Take steps immediately to relieve the obstruction. • If severe airway obstruction continues and the victim becomes unresponsive, start CPR. • If you are not alone, send someone to activate the emergency response system. If you are alone and must leave to activate the emergency response system, provide about 2 minutes of CPR before leaving.

Figure 40. The universal choking sign indicates the need for help when a victim is choking.

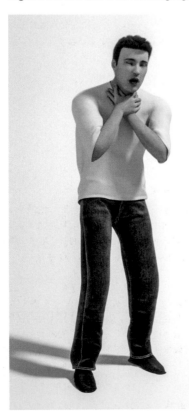

Choking Relief in a Responsive Adult or Child

Abdominal Thrusts

Use abdominal thrusts to relieve choking in a responsive adult or child. Do not use abdominal thrusts to relieve choking in an infant.

Give each individual thrust with the intention of relieving the obstruction. It may be necessary to repeat the thrust several times to clear the airway.

Abdominal Thrusts With the Victim Standing or Sitting

Follow these steps to perform abdominal thrusts on a responsive adult or child who is standing or sitting:

1. Stand or kneel behind the victim and wrap your arms around the victim's waist (Figure 41). Make a fist with one hand.
2. Place the thumb side of your fist against the victim's abdomen, in the midline, slightly above the navel and well below the breastbone.
3. Grasp your fist with your other hand and press your fist into the victim's abdomen with a quick, forceful upward thrust.
4. Repeat thrusts until the object is expelled from the airway or the victim becomes unresponsive.
5. Give each new thrust with a separate, distinct movement to relieve the obstruction.

Figure 41. Abdominal thrusts with the victim standing.

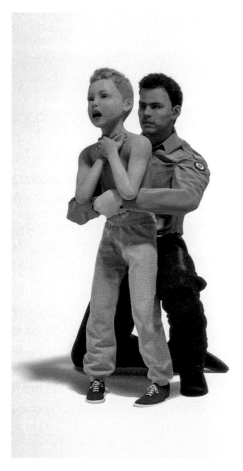

Choking Relief in Pregnant and Obese Victims

If the victim is pregnant or obese, perform chest thrusts instead of abdominal thrusts (Figure 42).

Figure 42. Perform chest thrusts instead of abdominal thrusts in a pregnant or obese choking victim.

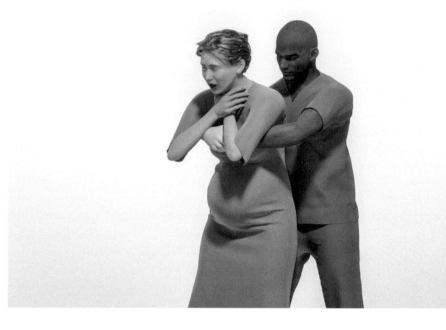

Choking Relief in an Unresponsive Adult or Child

A choking victim's condition may worsen, and the victim may become unresponsive. If you are aware that a foreign-body airway obstruction is causing the victim's condition, you will know to look for a foreign body in the throat.

To relieve choking in an unresponsive adult or child, follow these steps:

1. Shout for help. If someone else is available, send that person to activate the emergency response system.
2. Gently lower the victim to the ground if you see that they are becoming unresponsive.
3. Begin CPR, starting with chest compressions. Do not check for a pulse. Each time you open the airway to give breaths, open the victim's mouth wide. Look for the object.
   a. If you see an object that looks easy to remove, remove it with your fingers.
   b. If you do not see an object, continue CPR.
4. After about 5 cycles or 2 minutes of CPR, activate the emergency response system if someone has not already done so.

If a choking victim is already unresponsive when you arrive, you probably will not know if a foreign-body airway obstruction exists. In this situation, you should activate the emergency response system and start high-quality CPR.

Giving Effective Breaths When There Is an Airway Obstruction

When a choking victim loses consciousness, the muscles in the throat may relax. This could convert a complete/severe airway obstruction to a partial obstruction. In addition, chest compressions may create at least as much force as abdominal thrusts, so they may help expel the object. Giving 30 compressions and then removing any object that's visible in the mouth may allow you to eventually give effective breaths.

Actions After Choking Relief

You will know you successfully removed an airway obstruction in an unresponsive victim if you saw and removed a foreign body from the victim's mouth and the victim starts to breathe. However, you don't always have to remove the foreign body to successfully relieve the obstruction. If you can feel air movement and see the chest rise when you give breaths, the airway is no longer obstructed.

After you relieve choking in an unresponsive victim, proceed as you would with any unresponsive victim. Check again for responsiveness, check for breathing and a pulse, confirm that someone has activated the emergency response system, and provide high-quality CPR or rescue breathing as needed.

Encourage a *responsive* victim to seek immediate medical attention. A healthcare professional should evaluate the victim for potential complications from abdominal thrusts.

Choking Relief in Infants

Responsive Infant

Use back slaps and chest thrusts for choking relief in an infant. Do not use abdominal thrusts.

To relieve choking in a responsive infant, follow these steps:

1. Kneel or sit with the infant in your lap.
2. Hold the infant facedown with the head slightly lower than the chest, resting on your forearm. Support the infant's head and jaw with your hand. Take care to avoid compressing the soft tissues of the infant's throat. Rest your forearm on your lap or thigh to support the infant.
3. With the heel of your hand, deliver up to 5 forceful back slaps between the infant's shoulder blades (Figure 43A). Deliver each slap with enough force to attempt to dislodge the foreign body.
4. After delivering up to 5 back slaps, place your free hand on the infant's back, supporting the back of the infant's head with the palm of your hand. The infant will be adequately cradled between your 2 forearms, with the palm of one hand supporting the face and jaw while the palm of the other hand supports the back of the infant's head.
5. Turn the infant over while carefully supporting the head and neck. Hold the infant faceup, with your forearm resting on your thigh. Keep the infant's head lower than the trunk.
6. Provide up to 5 quick downward chest thrusts (Figure 43B) in the middle of the chest, over the lower half of the breastbone (the same location as for chest compressions during CPR). Deliver chest thrusts at a rate of about 1 per second, each with the intention of creating enough force to dislodge the foreign body.
7. Repeat the sequence of up to 5 back slaps and up to 5 chest thrusts until your actions have removed the object or the infant becomes unresponsive.

A

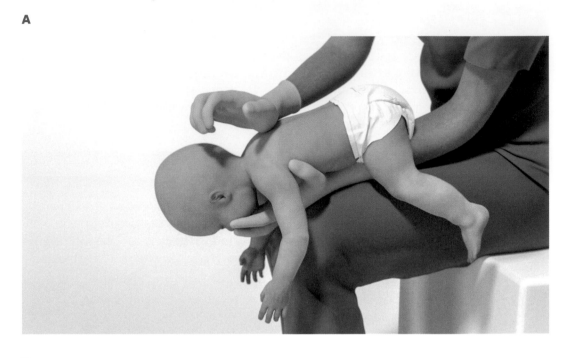

B

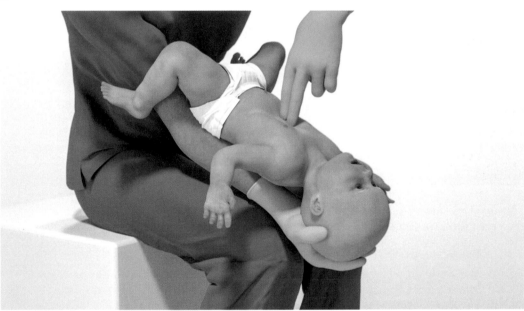

Unresponsive Infant

If the infant victim becomes unresponsive, stop giving back slaps and start CPR, starting with chest compressions.

To relieve choking in an unresponsive infant, follow these steps:

1. Shout for help. If someone responds, send that person to activate the emergency response system. Place the infant on a firm, flat surface.

2. Begin CPR (starting with compressions) with 1 extra step: Each time you open the airway, look for the object in the back of the throat. If you see an object and can easily remove it, remove it. Note that you do not check for a pulse before beginning CPR.

3. After about 2 minutes of CPR, activate the emergency response system (if no one has done so).

> ## Critical Concepts:
> ## No Blind Finger Sweeps

Do not perform a blind finger sweep because it may push the foreign body back into the airway, causing further obstruction or injury.

Review Questions

1. Which is an example of a mild foreign-body airway obstruction?
   a. Cyanosis (blue lips or skin)
   b. High-pitched noise while inhaling
   c. Inability to speak or cry
   d. Wheezing between coughs

2. Which victim of a severe airway obstruction should receive abdominal thrusts?
   a. An average-size 27-year-old man
   b. A woman who is obviously pregnant
   c. An obese 50-year-old man
   d. An average-size 9-month-old infant

3. You are performing abdominal thrusts on a 9-year-old child when she suddenly becomes unresponsive. After you shout for nearby help, what is the most appropriate action to take next?
   a. Begin high-quality CPR, starting with chest compressions.
   b. Check for a pulse.
   c. Continue performing abdominal thrusts.
   d. Provide 5 back slaps followed by 5 chest thrusts.

See Answers to Review Questions in the Appendix.

Appendix

Adult 1-Rescuer BLS Sequence

This is your step-by-step guide to providing high-quality CPR when you encounter an unresponsive adult and you are the only rescuer. The numbered steps correspond to the numbered steps on the Adult BLS Algorithm for Healthcare Providers (Figure 4 in Part 3).

The first rescuer who arrives at the side of a potential cardiac arrest victim should quickly perform Steps 1 and 2 and then begin high-quality CPR.

Step 1: Verify Scene Safety

Make sure that the scene is safe for you and the victim.

Step 2: Check for Responsiveness and Get Help

1. Tap the victim's shoulders and shout, "Are you OK?"
2. If the victim is not responsive, activate the emergency response system via mobile device. Get the AED or send someone to do so.

Step 3: Assess for Breathing and a Pulse

Next, assess the victim for normal breathing and a pulse (Figure 5) to determine next actions.

To minimize delay in starting CPR, you should assess breathing and pulse at the same time. This should take no more than 10 seconds.

For detailed instructions on checking for breathing and a pulse in an adult, see Part 3.

Steps 3a and 3b: Determine Next Actions

Determine next actions based on whether breathing is normal and if a pulse is felt.

- **If the victim is breathing normally and a pulse is felt,** monitor the victim until emergency responders arrive.
- **If the victim is not breathing normally but a pulse is felt:**
  - Provide rescue breathing at a rate of 1 breath every 6 seconds, or 10 breaths per minute (see Rescue Breathing in Part 8).
  - Check for a pulse about every 2 minutes. Perform high-quality CPR if you do not feel a pulse.
  - If you suspect opioid use, give naloxone if available and follow your local protocols (see Part 9 for more information).
- **If the victim is not breathing normally or is only gasping and has no pulse,** begin high-quality CPR (Step 4).

Step 4: Start High-Quality CPR

Start cycles of CPR with 30 chest compressions followed by 2 breaths (see Critical Concepts: High-Quality CPR in Part 1 and Perform High-Quality Chest Compressions in Part 3). Remove bulky clothing from the victim's chest so that you can locate appropriate hand placement for compressions. Removing the clothing will also aid in more rapid AED pad placement when the AED arrives.

Steps 5 and 6: Use the AED as Soon as It Is Available

Follow the AED directions to check the rhythm (see Part 4).

Step 7: If the AED Detects a Shockable Rhythm, Give a Shock

Give 1 shock. Resume CPR immediately until prompted by the AED to allow a rhythm check, about every 2 minutes. Continue CPR and using the AED until advanced life support providers take over or the victim begins to breathe, move, or otherwise react.

Step 8: If the AED Detects a Nonshockable Rhythm, Resume High-Quality CPR

Resume high-quality CPR until prompted by the AED to allow a rhythm check, about every 2 minutes. Continue CPR and using the AED until advanced life support providers take over or the victim begins to breathe, move, or otherwise react.

Adult 2-Rescuer BLS Sequence

This is your step-by-step guide to providing high-quality CPR to an unresponsive adult when you are part of a multirescuer (2 or more) team. The numbered steps correspond to the numbered steps on the Adult BLS Algorithm for Healthcare Providers (Figure 4 in Part 3). Follow the steps of the algorithm for the single rescuer; incorporation of additional rescuers is included here.

The first rescuer who arrives at the side of a potential cardiac arrest victim should quickly perform Steps 1 and 2 and then begin high-quality CPR. As more rescuers arrive, assign tasks (see Team Roles and Duties for 2 or More Rescuers in Part 3). When more rescuers are available for a resuscitation attempt, they can perform more tasks at the same time.

Step 1: Verify Scene Safety

Make sure the scene is safe for you and the victim.

Step 2: Check for Responsiveness and Get Help

1. Tap the victim's shoulders and shout, "Are you OK?"
2. If the victim is not responsive:
   a. The first rescuer assesses the victim and, if no mobile phone is available, sends the second rescuer to activate the emergency response system and retrieve the AED.

Step 3: Assess for Breathing and a Pulse

Next, assess the victim for normal breathing and a pulse (Figure 5) to determine next actions.

To minimize delay in starting CPR, you should assess breathing and pulse at the same time. This should take no more than 10 seconds.

For details, see Assess for Breathing and a Pulse in Part 3.

Steps 3a and 3b: Determine Next Actions

Determine next actions based on whether breathing is normal and if a pulse is felt:

- **If the victim is breathing normally and a pulse is felt,** monitor the victim.
- **If the victim is not breathing normally but a pulse is felt:**
  - Provide rescue breathing at a rate of 1 breath every 6 seconds, or 10 breaths per minute (see Rescue Breathing in Part 8).
  - Check for a pulse about every 2 minutes. Perform high-quality CPR if you do not feel a pulse.
  - If you suspect opioid use, give naloxone if available and follow your local protocols (see Part 9 for more information).
- **If the victim is not breathing normally or is only gasping and has no pulse,** begin high-quality CPR (Step 4).

Step 4: Begin High-Quality CPR, Starting With Chest Compressions

If the victim is not breathing normally or is only gasping and has no pulse, immediately do the following:

1. One rescuer begins high-quality CPR, starting with chest compressions. Remove bulky clothing from the victim's chest so that you can locate appropriate hand placement for compressions. Removing the clothing will also aid in more rapid AED pad placement when the AED arrives.
2. Once the second rescuer returns and assists in providing 2-rescuer CPR, switch compressors frequently (about every 2 minutes or 5 cycles, typically when the AED is analyzing the rhythm). This helps ensure that compressor fatigue does not reduce CPR quality (see Critical Concepts: High-Performance Teams in Part 3).

Steps 5 and 6: Use the AED as Soon as It Is Available

Follow the AED directions to check the rhythm (see Part 4).

Step 7: If the AED Detects a Shockable Rhythm, Give a Shock

Give 1 shock. Resume CPR immediately until prompted by the AED to allow a rhythm check, about every 2 minutes. Continue CPR and using the AED until more advanced life support providers take over or the victim begins to breathe, move, or otherwise react.

Step 8: If the AED Detects a Nonshockable Rhythm, Resume High-Quality CPR

Resume high-quality CPR until prompted by the AED to allow a rhythm check, about every 2 minutes. Continue CPR and using the AED until more advanced life support providers take over or the victim begins to breathe, move, or otherwise react.

Cardiac Arrest in Pregnancy: Out-of-Hospital BLS Considerations

This is your step-by-step guide to providing care for a pregnant victim in cardiac arrest. The steps correspond to the Adult BLS Algorithm for Healthcare Providers with specific pregnancy steps included. Goals of BLS with a pregnant victim include continuation of high-quality CPR with attention to good ventilation, continuous LUD, and rapid initiation of emergency services to determine proper transportation location and advanced care (Figure 44).

It is crucial to provide high-quality CPR for a pregnant woman just as you would for any victim of cardiac arrest. Without CPR, the lives of both the mother and the baby are at risk.

Figure 44. Adult BLS in Pregnancy Algorithm for Healthcare Providers.

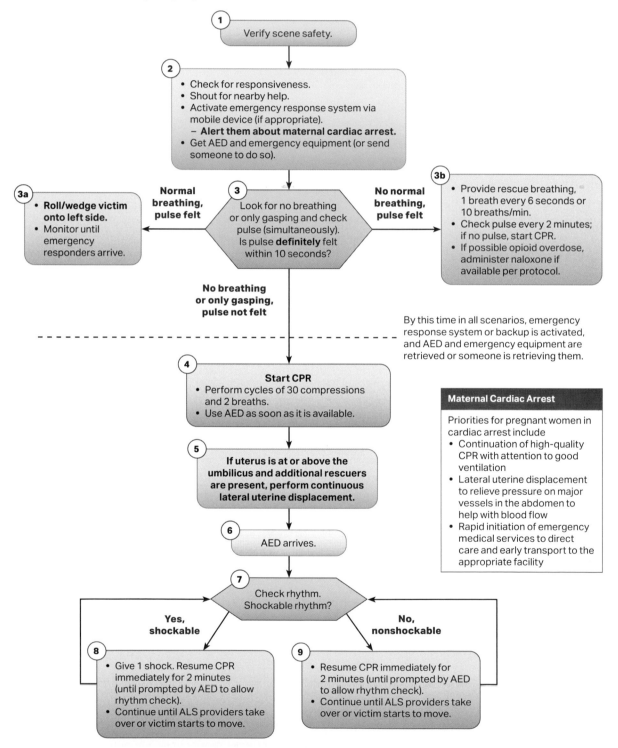

© 2020 American Heart Association

Rescuers who arrive at the side of a pregnant woman in cardiac arrest should follow these sequential steps on the algorithm:

Step 1: Verify Scene Safety

Make sure that the scene is safe for you and the victim.

Step 2: Check for Responsiveness and Get Help

1. Tap the victim's shoulders and shout, "Are you OK?"
2. If the victim is not responsive, activate the emergency response system via mobile device. Get the AED or send someone to do so.
3. Notify EMS of maternal arrest.

Step 3: Assess for Breathing and a Pulse

Next, assess the victim for normal breathing and a pulse (Figure 5) to determine next actions.

To minimize delay in starting CPR, you should assess breathing and pulse at the same time. This should take no more than 10 seconds.

For detailed instructions on checking for breathing and a pulse in an adult, see Part 3.

Steps 3a and 3b: Determine Next Actions

Determine next actions based on whether breathing is normal and if a pulse is felt.

- **If the victim is breathing normally and a pulse is felt,** monitor the victim until emergency responders arrive.

  - Roll or wedge the victim so that she is lying on her left side.

- **If the victim is not breathing normally but a pulse is felt:**
  - Provide rescue breathing at a rate of 1 breath every 6 seconds, or 10 breaths per minute (see Rescue Breathing in Part 8).
  - Check for a pulse about every 2 minutes. Perform high-quality CPR if you do not feel a pulse.
  - If you suspect opioid use, give naloxone if available and follow your local protocols (see Part 9 for more information).

- **If the victim is not breathing normally or is only gasping and has no pulse,** begin high-quality CPR (Step 4).

Step 4: Start High-Quality CPR

Start cycles of CPR with 30 chest compressions followed by 2 breaths (see Critical Concepts: High-Quality CPR in Part 1 and Perform High-Quality Chest Compressions in Part 3). Remove bulky clothing from the victim's chest so that you can locate appropriate hand placement for compressions. Removing the clothing will also aid in more rapid AED pad placement when the AED arrives. Use an AED as soon as it is available.

Step 5: LUD

If the uterus is at or above the umbilicus and additional rescuers are present, perform continuous LUD to relieve pressure on major vessels in the abdomen to help with blood flow (Figure 9).

- You should also provide LUD during rescue breathing if additional help is available.

Steps 6 and 7: Use the AED as Soon as It Is Available

Follow the AED directions to check the rhythm (see Part 4).

Step 8: If the AED Detects a Shockable Rhythm, Give a Shock

Give 1 shock. Resume CPR immediately until prompted by the AED to allow a rhythm check, about every 2 minutes. Continue CPR and using the AED until more advanced life support providers take over or the victim begins to breathe, move, or otherwise react.

Step 9: If the AED Detects a Nonshockable Rhythm, Resume High-Quality CPR

Resume high-quality CPR until prompted by the AED to allow a rhythm check, about every 2 minutes. Continue CPR and using the AED until more advanced life support providers take over or the victim begins to breathe, move, or otherwise react.

Opioid-Associated Emergency for Healthcare Providers Algorithm and Sequence

This is your step-by-step guide to providing care for a victim with a suspected opioid-associated emergency. The numbered steps correspond to the numbered boxes on the Opioid-Associated Emergency for Healthcare Providers Algorithm (Figure 45). As with all emergency situations begin by assessing the scene for your safety and the safety of the victim.

Figure 45. Opioid-Associated Emergency for Healthcare Providers Algorithm.

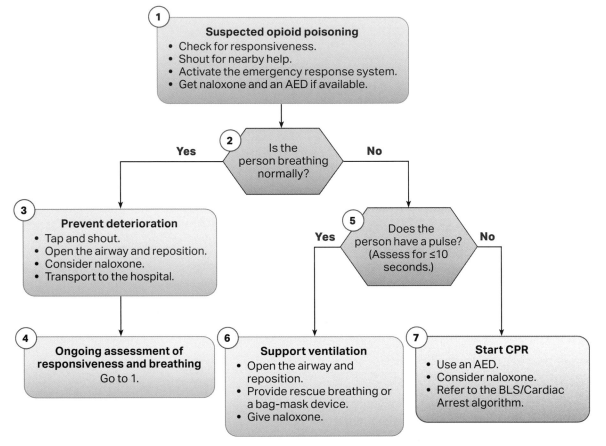

© 2020 American Heart Association

The first rescuer who arrives at the side of someone who has a suspected opioid-associated emergency should follow these sequential steps on the algorithm:

Step 1: Suspect Opioid Poisoning

- Check to see if the person responds.
- Shout for nearby help.
- Activate the emergency response system.
- If you are alone, get naloxone and an AED if available. If someone else is present, send that person to get them.

Step 2: Is the Person Breathing Normally?

- If the person is breathing normally, proceed with Steps 3 and 4.
- If the person is not breathing normally, go to Step 5.

Step 3: Prevent Deterioration

- Tap and shout. Check for responsiveness by tapping the victim's shoulders. Shout, "Are you OK?"
- Open and reposition the airway if needed to maintain normal breathing. This may be necessary if the victim is unresponsive or is responsive but unable to maintain an open airway due to a depressed level of consciousness.
- Consider administering naloxone, if available. If you suspect an opioid overdose, it is reasonable to give naloxone according to package directions and per local protocol. Monitor for response.
- Transport to the hospital. If the victim is not already in a healthcare setting, they should be transported by EMS to a hospital.

Step 4: Assess for Responsiveness and Breathing

Continue to assess responsiveness and breathing until the victim is transferred to advanced care. Victims with opioid-associated emergencies may not be able to maintain an open airway or breathe normally. Even those who receive naloxone may develop respiratory problems that can lead to cardiac arrest.

Step 5: Does the Person Have a Pulse?

Assess for a pulse for no more than 10 seconds.

- If yes (a pulse is felt), go to Step 6.
- If no (a pulse is not felt), go to Step 7.

Step 6: Support Ventilation

- Open and reposition the airway before giving rescue breaths.
- Provide rescue breathing or bag-mask ventilation. This can help prevent cardiac arrest. Continue until spontaneous, normal breathing occurs. Reassess the victim's breathing and pulse every 2 minutes. If there is no pulse, provide CPR (see Step 7).
- Give naloxone according to package directions and per local protocol.

Step 7: Start CPR

- If the victim is not breathing normally and no pulse is felt, provide high-quality CPR, including ventilation. Use the AED as soon as it is available.
- Consider naloxone. If naloxone is available and you suspect an opioid overdose, it is reasonable to give it according to package directions and per local protocol. High-quality CPR should take priority over giving naloxone.
- Refer to the BLS protocol (see Figure 4).

Infant and Child 1-Rescuer BLS Sequence

This is your step-by-step guide to providing CPR to an unresponsive infant or child when you are the only rescuer. The numbered steps correspond to the numbered steps on the Pediatric BLS Algorithm for Healthcare Providers—Single Rescuer (Figure 27 in Part 6).

The first rescuer who arrives at the side of an unresponsive infant or child should quickly perform Steps 1 and 2 and then begin high-quality CPR.

Step 1: Verify Scene Safety

Make sure the scene is safe for you and the victim.

Step 2: Check for Responsiveness and Get Help

1. Tap the child's shoulders. Shout, "Are you OK?"
2. If the victim is not responsive, shout for help and activate the emergency response system via mobile device if appropriate.

Step 3: Assess for Breathing and a Pulse

Next, assess the infant or child for normal breathing and a pulse. This will help you determine the next appropriate actions.

To minimize delay in starting CPR, you should assess breathing and pulse at the same time. This should take no more than 10 seconds.

For detailed instructions on checking for breathing and a pulse in an infant and in a child, see High-Quality CPR Skills: Infants and Children in Part 6.

Steps 3a and 3b: Determine Next Actions

Determine next actions based on the presence or absence of normal breathing and a pulse:

- **If the victim is breathing normally and a pulse is felt:**
  - Activate the emergency response system (if not already done).
  - Monitor the victim until emergency responders arrive.
- **If the victim is not breathing normally but a pulse is felt:**
  - Provide rescue breathing, with 1 breath every 2 to 3 seconds, or 20 to 30 breaths per minute.
  - Assess the pulse rate for 10 seconds.

Steps 4, 4a, and 4b: Is the Heart Rate Less Than 60/Min With Signs of Poor Perfusion?

- If yes, start CPR.
- If no, continue rescue breathing. Check for a pulse about every 2 minutes. If no pulse, start CPR.

Steps 5 and 5a: Was the Sudden Collapse Witnessed?

If yes, activate the emergency response system (if not already done), and get the AED.

Step 6: If the Collapse Was Not Witnessed:

Start CPR with cycles of 30 compressions and 2 breaths. Remove bulky clothing from the victim's chest so that you can locate appropriate hand or finger placement for compression. Removing the clothing will also aid in more rapid AED pad placement when the AED arrives. Use the AED as soon as it is available.

Single rescuers should use the following compression techniques (see Perform High-Quality Chest Compressions in Part 6 for complete details):

- For an infant, use either the 2-finger or 2 thumb–encircling hands technique
- For a child, use 1 or 2 hands (whatever is needed to provide compressions of adequate depth)

Step 7: Activate the Emergency Response System and Get an AED

After about 2 minutes, if you are still alone, activate the emergency response system and get an AED if not already done.

Step 8: Use the AED as Soon as It Is Available

Follow the AED directions to check the rhythm.

Step 9: If the AED Detects a Shockable Rhythm, Give 1 Shock

Give a shock. Resume CPR immediately until prompted by the AED to allow a rhythm check, about every 2 minutes. Continue CPR and using the AED until advanced life support providers take over or the victim begins to breathe, move, or otherwise react.

Step 10: If the AED Detects a Nonshockable Rhythm, Resume High-Quality CPR

Resume high-quality CPR until prompted by the AED to allow a rhythm check, about every 2 minutes. Continue CPR and using the AED until advanced life support providers take over or the victim begins to breathe, move, or otherwise react.

Infant and Child 2-Rescuer BLS Sequence

This is your step-by-step guide to providing CPR to an unresponsive infant or child when you are part of a multirescuer (2 or more) team. The numbered steps correspond to the numbered steps on the Pediatric BLS Algorithm for Healthcare Providers—2 or More Rescuers (Figure 31 in Part 6).

The first rescuer who arrives at the side of an unresponsive infant or child should quickly perform Steps 1 and 2. As more rescuers arrive, assign roles and responsibilities. When more rescuers are available for a resuscitation attempt, they can perform more tasks at the same time.

Step 1: Verify Scene Safety

Make sure that the scene is safe for you and the victim.

Step 2: Check for Responsiveness and Get Help

1. Tap the child's shoulders. Shout, "Are you OK?"
2. If the victim is not responsive, shout for help and activate the emergency response via mobile device if appropriate.
3. The first rescuer remains with the victim while the second rescuer activates the emergency response system and retrieves the AED and emergency equipment (Figure 46).

Figure 46. If the arrest of an infant or child was sudden and witnessed, activate the emergency response system in your setting. **A,** In-facility setting. **B,** Prehospital setting.

A   **B**

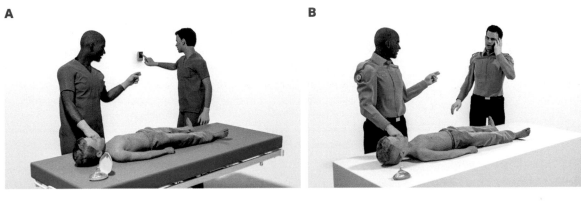

Step 3: Assess for Breathing and a Pulse

Next, assess the infant or child for normal breathing and a pulse. This will help you determine the next appropriate actions.

To minimize delay in starting CPR, you should assess breathing and pulse at the same time. This should take no more than 10 seconds.

For detailed instructions on checking for breathing and a pulse in an infant and in a child, see High-Quality CPR Skills: Infants and Children in Part 6.

Steps 3a and 3b: Determine Next Actions

Determine next action based on whether breathing is normal and if a pulse is felt:

- **If the victim is breathing normally and a pulse is felt,** activate the emergency response system. Monitor the victim until emergency responders arrive.
- **If the victim is not breathing normally but a pulse is felt:**
  - Provide rescue breathing, with 1 breath every 2 to 3 seconds, or 20 to 30 breaths per minute.
  - Assess the pulse rate for 10 seconds.

Steps 4, 4a, and 4b: Is the Heart Rate Less Than 60/Min With Signs of Poor Perfusion?

- If yes, start CPR.
- If no, continue rescue breathing. Check for a pulse about every 2 minutes. If no pulse, start CPR.

Step 5: Begin High-Quality CPR, Starting With Chest Compressions

- The first rescuer starts cycles of CPR with 30 compressions and 2 breaths. When the second rescuer returns, continue cycles of CPR with 15 compressions and 2 breaths. Remove bulky clothing from the victim's chest so that you can locate appropriate hand or finger placement for compression. Removing the clothing will also aid in more rapid AED pad placement when the AED arrives. Use the AED as soon as it is available.
  - For an infant, use either the 2-finger or 2 thumb–encircling hands technique until the second rescuer returns to provide 2-rescuer CPR. During 2-rescuer CPR, the 2 thumb–encircling hands technique is preferred. (See Perform High-Quality Chest Compressions in Part 6 for instructions on both techniques.)
  - For a child, use 1 or 2 hands (1 hand for a very small child).
- When the second rescuer returns, that rescuer gives breaths.
- Rescuers should switch compressors about every 2 minutes (or earlier if needed) so that compressor fatigue does not reduce CPR quality (see Critical Concepts: High-Performance Teams in Part 3).

Step 6: Prepare for Defibrillation With the AED

Follow the AED directions to check the rhythm.

Step 7: If the AED Detects a Shockable Rhythm, Give 1 Shock.

Give a shock. Resume CPR immediately until prompted by the AED to allow a rhythm check, about every 2 minutes. Continue CPR and using the AED until advanced life support providers take over or the victim begins to breathe, move, or otherwise react.

Step 8: If the AED Detects a Shockable Rhythm, Resume High-Quality CPR

Resume high-quality CPR until prompted by the AED to allow a rhythm check, about every 2 minutes. Continue CPR and using the AED until advanced providers take over or the victim begins to breathe, move, or otherwise react.

Summary of High-Quality CPR Components for BLS Providers

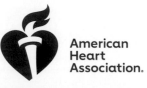
American Heart Association.

Component	Adults and adolescents	Children (age 1 year to puberty)	Infants (age less than 1 year, excluding newborns)
Verifying scene safety	Make sure the environment is safe for rescuers and victim		
Recognizing cardiac arrest	Check for responsiveness No breathing or only gasping (ie, no normal breathing) No definite pulse felt within 10 seconds (Breathing and pulse check can be performed simultaneously in less than 10 seconds)		
Activating emergency response system	*If a mobile device is available, phone emergency services (9-1-1)*		
	If you are alone with no mobile phone, leave the victim to activate the emergency response system and get the AED before beginning CPR Otherwise, send someone and begin CPR immediately; use the AED as soon as it is available	*Witnessed collapse* Follow steps for adults and adolescents on the left *Unwitnessed collapse* Give 2 minutes of CPR Leave the victim to activate the emergency response system and get the AED Return to the child or infant and resume CPR; use the AED as soon as it is available	
Compression-ventilation ratio *without advanced airway*	*1 or 2 rescuers* 30:2	*1 rescuer* 30:2 *2 or more rescuers* 15:2	
Compression-ventilation ratio *with advanced airway*	Continuous compressions at a rate of 100-120/min Give 1 breath every 6 seconds (10 breaths/min)	Continuous compressions at a rate of 100-120/min Give 1 breath every 2-3 seconds (20-30 breaths/min)	
Compression rate	100-120/min		
Compression depth	At least 2 inches (5 cm)*	At least one third AP diameter of chest Approximately 2 inches (5 cm)	At least one third AP diameter of chest Approximately 1½ inches (4 cm)
Hand placement	2 hands on the lower half of the breastbone (sternum)	2 hands or 1 hand (optional for very small child) on the lower half of the breastbone (sternum)	*1 rescuer* 2 fingers or 2 thumbs in the center of the chest, just below the nipple line *2 or more rescuers* 2 thumb–encircling hands in the center of the chest, just below the nipple line If the rescuer is unable to achieve the recommended depth, it may be reasonable to use the heel of one hand
Chest recoil	Allow complete recoil of chest after each compression; do not lean on the chest after each compression		
Minimizing interruptions	Limit interruptions in chest compressions to less than 10 seconds with a CCF goal of 80%		

*Compression depth should be no more than 2.4 inches (6 cm).
Abbreviations: AED, automated external defibrillator; AP, anteroposterior; CCF, chest compression fraction; CPR, cardiopulmonary resuscitation.

© 2020 American Heart Association

Basic Life Support
Adult CPR and AED
Skills Testing Checklist

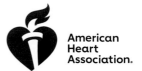
American Heart Association.

Student Name _____ Date of Test _____

Hospital Scenario: "You are working in a hospital or clinic, and you see a person who has suddenly collapsed in the hallway. You check that the scene is safe and then approach the patient. Demonstrate what you would do next."

Prehospital Scenario: "You arrive on the scene for a suspected cardiac arrest. No bystander CPR has been provided. You approach the scene and ensure that it is safe. Demonstrate what you would do next."

Assessment and Activation

☐ Checks responsiveness   ☐ Shouts for help/Activates emergency response system/Sends for AED

☐ Checks breathing   ☐ Checks pulse

Once student shouts for help, instructor says, "Here's the barrier device. I am going to get the AED."

Cycle 1 of CPR (30:2)   **CPR feedback devices are required for accuracy*

Adult Compressions

☐ Performs high-quality compressions*:

• Hand placement on lower half of sternum

• 30 compressions in no less than 15 and no more than 18 seconds

• Compresses at least 2 inches (5 cm)

• Complete recoil after each compression

Adult Breaths

☐ Gives 2 breaths with a barrier device:

• Each breath given over 1 second

• Visible chest rise with each breath

• Resumes compressions in less than 10 seconds

Cycle 2 of CPR (repeats steps in Cycle 1)   *Only check box if step is successfully performed*

☐ Compressions   ☐ Breaths   ☐ Resumes compressions in less than 10 seconds

---

Rescuer 2 says, "Here is the AED. I'll take over compressions, and you use the AED."

AED (follows prompts of AED)

☐ Powers on AED   ☐ Correctly attaches pads   ☐ Clears for analysis

☐ Clears to safely deliver a shock   ☐ Safely delivers a shock

---

Resumes Compressions

☐ Ensures compressions are resumed immediately after shock delivery

• Student directs instructor to resume compressions *or*

• Second student resumes compressions

STOP TEST

Instructor Notes

• Place a check in the box next to each step the student completes successfully.

• If the student does not complete all steps successfully (as indicated by at least 1 blank check box), the student must receive remediation. Make a note here of which skills require remediation (refer to instructor manual for information about remediation).

Test Results Circle **PASS** or **NR** to indicate pass or needs remediation:	**PASS**	**NR**

Instructor Initials _____   Instructor Number _____   Date _____

Basic Life Support
Adult CPR and AED
Skills Testing Critical Skills Descriptors

1. **Assesses victim and activates emergency response system (this _must_ precede starting compressions) within 30 seconds. After determining that the scene is safe:**
   - Checks for responsiveness by tapping and shouting
   - Shouts for help/directs someone to call for help _and_ get AED/defibrillator
   - Checks for no breathing or no normal breathing (only gasping)
     - Scans from the head to the chest for a minimum of 5 seconds and no more than 10 seconds
   - Checks carotid pulse
     - Can be done simultaneously with check for breathing
     - Checks for a minimum of 5 seconds and no more than 10 seconds
2. **Performs high-quality chest compressions (initiates compressions immediately after recognition of cardiac arrest)**
   - Correct hand placement
     - Lower half of sternum
     - 2-handed (second hand on top of the first or grasping the wrist of the first hand)
   - Compression rate of 100 to 120/min
     - Delivers 30 compressions in 15 to 18 seconds
   - Compression depth and recoil—at least 2 inches (5 cm) and avoid compressing more than 2.4 inches (6 cm)
     - Use of a commercial feedback device or high-fidelity manikin is required
     - Complete chest recoil after each compression
   - Minimizes interruptions in compressions
     - Delivers 2 breaths so less than 10 seconds elapses between last compression of one cycle and first compression of next cycle
     - Compressions resumed immediately after shock/no shock indicated
3. **Provides 2 breaths by using a barrier device**
   - Opens airway adequately
     - Uses a head tilt–chin lift maneuver or jaw thrust
   - Delivers each breath over 1 second
   - Delivers breaths that produce visible chest rise
   - Avoids excessive ventilation
   - Resumes chest compressions in less than 10 seconds
4. **Performs same steps for compressions and breaths for Cycle 2**
5. **AED use**
   - Powers on AED
     - Turns AED on by pushing button or lifting lid as soon as it arrives
   - Correctly attaches pads
     - Places proper-sized (adult) pads for victim's age in correct location
   - Clears for analysis
     - Clears rescuers from victim for AED to analyze rhythm (pushes analyze button if required by device)
     - Communicates clearly to all other rescuers to stop touching victim
   - Clears to safely deliver shock
     - Communicates clearly to all other rescuers to stop touching victim
   - Safely delivers a shock
     - Resumes chest compressions immediately after shock delivery
     - Does not turn off AED during CPR
6. **Resumes compressions**
   - Ensures that high-quality chest compressions are resumed immediately after shock delivery
     - Performs same steps for compressions

Infant CPR
Skills Testing Checklist (1 of 2)

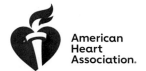

American Heart Association.

Student Name _____   Date of Test _____

Hospital Scenario: "You are working in a hospital or clinic when a woman runs through the door, carrying an infant. She shouts, 'Help me! My baby's not breathing.' You have gloves and a pocket mask. You send your coworker to activate the emergency response system and to get the emergency equipment."

Prehospital Scenario: "You arrive on the scene for an infant who is not breathing. No bystander CPR has been provided. You approach the scene and ensure that it is safe. Demonstrate what you would do next."

Assessment and Activation
- ☐ Checks responsiveness
- ☐ Checks breathing
- ☐ Shouts for help/Activates emergency response system
- ☐ Checks pulse

Once student shouts for help, instructor says, "Here's the barrier device."

Cycle 1 of CPR (30:2)   **CPR feedback devices are preferred for accuracy*
Infant Compressions
- ☐ Performs high-quality compressions*:
  - Placement of 2 fingers or 2 thumbs in the center of the chest, just below the nipple line
  - 30 compressions in no less than 15 and no more than 18 seconds
  - Compresses at least one third the depth of the chest, approximately 1½ inches (4 cm)
  - Complete recoil after each compression

Infant Breaths
- ☐ Gives 2 breaths with a barrier device:
  - Each breath given over 1 second
  - Visible chest rise with each breath
  - Resumes compressions in less than 10 seconds

Cycle 2 of CPR (repeats steps in Cycle 1)   *Only check box if step is successfully performed*
- ☐ Compressions   ☐ Breaths   ☐ Resumes compressions in less than 10 seconds

---

Rescuer 2 arrives with bag-mask device and begins ventilation while Rescuer 1 continues compressions with 2 thumb–encircling hands technique.

Cycle 3 of CPR
Rescuer 1: Infant Compressions
- ☐ Performs high-quality compressions*:
  - 15 compressions with 2 thumb–encircling hands technique
  - 15 compressions in no less than 7 and no more than 9 seconds
  - Compresses at least one third the depth of the chest, approximately 1½ inches (4 cm)
  - Complete recoil after each compression

Rescuer 2: Infant Breaths
This rescuer is not evaluated.

(continued)

Infant CPR
Skills Testing Checklist (2 of 2)

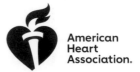

American
Heart
Association.

Student Name _____   Date of Test _____

(continued)

Cycle 4 of CPR

Rescuer 2: Infant Compressions

This rescuer is not evaluated.

Rescuer 1: Infant Breaths

☐ Gives 2 breaths with a bag-mask device:

• Each breath given over 1 second

• Visible chest rise with each breath

• Resumes compressions in less than 10 seconds

STOP TEST

Instructor Notes
• Place a check in the box next to each step the student completes successfully.
• If the student does not complete all steps successfully (as indicated by at least 1 blank check box), the student must receive remediation. Make a note here of which skills require remediation (refer to instructor manual for information about remediation).

Test Results	Circle **PASS** or **NR** to indicate pass or needs remediation:	**PASS**	**NR**

Instructor Initials _____   Instructor Number _____   Date _____

Basic Life Support
Infant CPR
Skills Testing Critical Skills Descriptors

1. **Assesses victim and activates emergency response system (this *must* precede starting compressions) within 30 seconds. After determining that the scene is safe:**
   - Checks for responsiveness by tapping and shouting
   - Shouts for help/directs someone to call for help *and* get emergency equipment
   - Checks for no breathing or no normal breathing (only gasping)
     - Scans from the head to the chest for a minimum of 5 seconds and no more than 10 seconds
   - Checks brachial pulse
     - Can be done simultaneously with check for breathing
     - Checks for a minimum of 5 seconds and no more than 10 seconds

2. **Performs high-quality chest compressions during 1-rescuer CPR (initiates compressions within 10 seconds after identifying cardiac arrest)**
   - Correct placement of hands/fingers in center of chest
     - 1 rescuer: 2 fingers or 2 thumbs just below the nipple line
     - *If the rescuer is unable to achieve the recommended depth, it may be reasonable to use the heel of one hand*
   - Compression rate of 100 to 120/min
     - Delivers 30 compressions in 15 to 18 seconds
   - Adequate depth for age
     - Infant: at least one third the depth of the chest (approximately 1½ inches [4 cm])
     - Use of a commercial feedback device or high-fidelity manikin is preferred
   - Complete chest recoil after each compression
   - Appropriate ratio for age and number of rescuers
     - 1 rescuer: 30 compressions to 2 breaths
   - Minimizes interruptions in compressions
     - Delivers 2 breaths so less than 10 seconds elapses between last compression of one cycle and first compression of next cycle

3. **Provides effective breaths with bag-mask device during 2-rescuer CPR**
   - Opens airway adequately
   - Delivers each breath over 1 second
   - Delivers breaths that produce visible chest rise
   - Avoids excessive ventilation
   - Resumes chest compressions in less than 10 seconds

4. **Switches compression technique at appropriate interval as prompted by the instructor (for purposes of this evaluation). Switch should take no more than 5 seconds.**

5. **Performs high-quality chest compressions during 2-rescuer CPR**
   - Correct placement of hands/fingers in center of chest
     - 2 rescuers: 2 thumb–encircling hands just below the nipple line
   - Compression rate of 100 to 120/min
     - Delivers 15 compressions in 7 to 9 seconds
   - Adequate depth for age
     - Infant: at least one third the depth of the chest (approximately 1½ inches [4 cm])
   - Complete chest recoil after each compression
   - Appropriate ratio for age and number of rescuers
     - 2 rescuers: 15 compressions to 2 breaths
   - Minimizes interruptions in compressions
   - Delivers 2 breaths so less than 10 seconds elapses between last compression of one cycle and first compression of next cycle

Glossary

30:2 CPR: CPR that is provided in a ratio of 30 chest compressions to 2 breaths.

Abdominal thrusts: A procedure used to force a foreign object from a choking victim's airway; sometimes called the *Heimlich maneuver.*

Adult and adolescent: Anyone with visible signs of puberty (chest or underarm hair in males; any breast development in females) and older.

Agonal gasps: An abnormal, reflexive breathing pattern that may be present in the first minutes after sudden cardiac arrest. The victim with agonal gasps appears to be drawing in air very quickly. Gasps happen at a slow rate. They may sound like a snort, snore, or groan. Agonal gasps are not normal breathing and do not provide adequate oxygenation and ventilation.

Arrhythmia: An irregular rhythm or abnormal heartbeat; occurs when the electrical impulses that cause the heart to beat happen too quickly, too slowly, or erratically.

Automated external defibrillator (AED): A lightweight, portable, computerized device that can identify an abnormal heart rhythm that may need a shock. If the AED identifies a shockable rhythm, it then can deliver an electrical shock through pads placed on the cardiac arrest victim's chest. The shock can reset an abnormal heart rhythm.

AEDs are simple to operate. Laypeople and healthcare providers can provide defibrillation safely by following the AED's visual or audible prompts.

Bag-mask device: A hand-held device consisting of an inflatable bag attached to a face mask; used to provide effective ventilation to a victim with ineffective or absent breathing. A bag-mask device may be used with or without supplemental oxygen.

Cardiac arrest: The abrupt loss of heart function in a person who may or may not have been diagnosed with heart disease. It can come on suddenly or in the wake of other symptoms. Cardiac arrest is often fatal if appropriate steps aren't taken immediately.

Cardiac catheterization procedure: A procedure that uses diagnostic imaging equipment to evaluate blood flow in and through the heart. During the procedure, a catheter is inserted in an artery (most frequently the groin or wrist) and threaded through the blood vessels to the patient's heart so that providers can visualize the arteries and chambers of the heart. Some cardiac problems, such as a blocked artery or other abnormalities, can be treated during the procedure. The procedure is performed in a cardiac catherization suite, also called a *cath lab.*

Cardiopulmonary resuscitation (CPR): A lifesaving emergency procedure for a victim who has signs of cardiac arrest (ie, unresponsive, no normal breathing, and no pulse). The 2 key components of CPR are chest compressions and breaths.

Chest compression fraction (CCF): The proportion of time that rescuers perform chest compressions during CPR. A CCF of at least 60% increases the likelihood of return of spontaneous circulation and survival to hospital discharge. With good teamwork, rescuers often can achieve 80% or greater.

Chest recoil: When the chest reexpands and comes back up to its normal position after a chest compression.

Child: 1 year of age to puberty (signs of puberty are chest or underarm hair in males; any breast development in females).

Defibrillation: Interrupting or stopping an abnormal heart rhythm by using controlled electrical shocks.

Gastric inflation (gastric distention): When the stomach fills with air during CPR; it is more likely to occur when the victim's airway isn't positioned properly, and air from ventilation goes into the stomach instead of the lungs. Another cause is when rescuers give breaths too quickly or too forcefully. Gastric inflation often interferes with properly ventilating the lungs. It also can cause vomiting.

Hands-Only CPR: Providing chest compressions without rescue breathing during CPR.

Head tilt–chin lift: A maneuver used to open a victim's airway before providing rescue breaths during CPR.

Heart attack: When a blockage or spasm occurs in a blood vessel and severely restricts or cuts off the flow of blood and oxygen to the heart muscle. During a heart attack, the heart typically continues to pump blood. But the longer the person with a heart attack goes without treatment to restore blood flow, the greater the possible damage to the heart muscle.

In-hospital cardiac arrest: A cardiac arrest that occurs inside a hospital.

Infant: A child younger than 1 year of age (excluding newly born infants in the delivery room).

Jaw thrust: A maneuver used to open a victim's airway before providing rescue breaths during CPR; used when the victim may have a spinal injury or when a head tilt–chin lift doesn't work.

Lateral uterine displacement: The process of using 1 or 2 hands to manually move the visibly pregnant abdomen of a woman to the left side by either pushing or pulling. This action will move the baby off of the large blood vessels that run from the lower body to the heart and help to improve blood flow provided by CPR.

Naloxone: An antidote that partially or completely reverses the effects of an opioid overdose, including respiratory depression. This medication may be given via several routes. The most common routes for emergency use in patients with known or suspected opioid overdose are intramuscularly by autoinjector or intranasally via nasal atomizer device.

Out-of-hospital cardiac arrest: A cardiac arrest that occurs outside of a hospital.

Opioids: A class of drugs that produces narcotic effects of pain relief; includes prescription drugs (hydrocodone, fentanyl, morphine) and illegal drugs (heroin). Misuse or overuse can cause respiratory depression and lead to cardiac arrest.

Personal protective equipment (PPE): Equipment such as protective clothing, helmets, and goggles designed to protect the wearer's body from injury or infection. Some hazards addressed by PPE are airborne particulate matter, physical hazards, chemicals, and biohazards. Common PPE for healthcare providers includes gloves, eye covering, masks, and gowns.

Pocket mask: A handheld device consisting of a face mask with a 1-way valve; the rescuer places it over a victim's nose and mouth as a barrier device when giving rescue breaths during CPR.

Public access defibrillation (PAD): Having AEDs available in public places where large numbers of people gather, such as airports, office buildings, and schools, or where there are people at high risk for heart attacks. Programs may also include CPR and AED training for potential rescuers and coordination with local EMS.

Pulseless ventricular tachycardia (pVT): A life-threatening shockable cardiac rhythm that results in ineffective ventricular contractions. The rapid quivering of the ventricular walls prevents them from pumping so that pulses are not detectable (ie, the "pulseless" in pVT). Body tissues and organs, especially the heart and brain, no longer receive oxygen.

Respiratory arrest: A life-threatening emergency that occurs when normal breathing stops or when breathing is not effective. If untreated, it will lead to cardiac arrest, or it can occur at the same time as cardiac arrest.

Return of spontaneous circulation (ROSC): When a victim of cardiac arrest resumes a sustained heartbeat that produces palpable pulses. Signs of ROSC include breathing, coughing, or movement and a palpable pulse or measurable blood pressure.

Shock: A life-threatening condition that occurs when the circulatory system can't maintain adequate blood flow; the delivery of oxygen and nutrients to vital tissues and organs is sharply reduced.

Telecommunicator CPR (T-CPR): Live, instant instructions provided over the phone by a telecommunicator (eg, dispatcher or emergency call taker) to a 9-1-1 caller. The telecommunicator helps the rescuer recognize a cardiac arrest and coaches them in how to provide effective CPR. For example, T-CPR assists the untrained rescuer in performing high-quality compression-only CPR. T-CPR coaches the trained rescuer in performing high-quality 30:2 CPR.

Ventricular fibrillation: A life-threatening shockable cardiac rhythm that results when the heart's electrical activity becomes chaotic. The heart muscles quiver in a fast, unsynchronized way so that the heart does not pump blood.

Answers to Review Questions

Part 1: [No review questions]

Part 2: 1.b, 2.c, 3.d

Part 3: 1.d, 2.d, 3.a, 4.c, 5.d, 6.a, 7.b, 8.c

Part 4: 1.c, 2.b, 3.a, 4.d

Part 5: 1.c, 2.c, 3.a

Part 6: 1.d, 2.b, 3.d, 4.c, 5.b

Part 7: 1.c, 2.b, 3.c

Part 8: 1.c, 2.a, 3.a, 4.b

Part 9: 1.d, 2.c, 3.b

Part 10: 1.b, 2.a, 3.d, 4.b, 5.c, 6.d, 7.b, 8.a

Part 11: 1.d, 2.a, 3.a

Recommended Reading

2020 Handbook of Emergency Cardiovascular Care for Healthcare Providers. Dallas, TX: American Heart Association; 2020.

American Heart Association. American Heart Association Guidelines for CPR and ECC. Web-based integrated guidelines site. ECCguidelines.heart.org. Originally published October 2020.

Highlights of the 2020 American Heart Association Guidelines for CPR and ECC. Dallas, TX: American Heart Association; 2020. ECCguidelines.heart.org.